Intermittent Fasting for Women Over 50

The Complete Guide to Lose Weight for Aging Women. How to Start a New Lifestyle, Detox your Body and Improve the Quality of your Life with Autophagy.

© Copyright 2020 - All rights reserved.

Table of Contents

Introduction **6**

Chapter 1: What Is Intermittent Fasting? **8**

Chapter 2: How Intermittent Fasting Works **17**

Two IF States: Fed Vs. Fasted 19

Chapter 3: Is Intermittent Fasting Good For Women? 21

Advantages Of Intermittent Fasting 23

Disadvantages Of Intermittent Fasting 27

Chapter 4: The Differences Between The Young Vs Older Woman **35**

Differences Between The Young Vs. Older Woman 37

How IF Affects Women At This Age And How To Approach It 39

Anti-Aging Foods 40

Tips And Exercises To Lose Belly Fat And Kickstart Your Metabolism 47

Best (IF) Methods For Health And Weight Loss At This Age 48

Chapter 5: How Intermittent Fasting Affects Women At This Age And How To Approach It **51**

Intermittent Fasting For The Weight Loss Process 53

Intermittent Fasting For Preventing Diseases 55

Intermittent Fasting For The Anti-Aging Process 55

Intermittent Fasting Practiced For Therapeutic Benefits 57

Intermittent Fasting For Better Mental Performance 58

Intermittent Fasting For An Improved Physical Fitness 58

Intermittent Fasting For Bodybuilding 61

Chapter 6: Intermittent Fasting Types **63**

Explanation Of Different Methods 64

Lean-Gains Method 64

16:8 Method 65

14:10 Method 66

20:4 Method 67

The Warrior Method 68

12:12 Method 69

5:2 Method 69

Eat-Stop-Eat (24-Hour) Method 70

Alternate-Day Method 72

Spontaneous Skipping Method 73

Crescendo Method 74

Making Your Choice 76

Chapter 7: What To Eat.................................. **82**

Chapter 8: Commons Mistakes And How To Fix Them
....**87**

Busting The Myths.....................................*87*

Common Intermittent Fasting Mistakes To Avoid..............*88*

Chapter 9: Intermittent Fasting Tips **97**

Transitional Tips *98*

Help For Routine-Setting *100*

What To Expect.......................................*100*

What To Do/What Not To Do.............................*103*

What To Lookout For..................................*106*

When To Quit *107*

Chapter 10: Why Intermittent Fasting Is Ideal For Women Over 50..**109**

Chapter 11: Life-Changing Tips For Weight Loss Success...**126**

Chapter 12: Mostly Asked Questions And Answers On Intermittent Fasting **140**

Conclusion **150**

Introduction

Being over 50 and a woman trying to lose weight and get healthier is not an easy task. So much seems impossible to do like going to the gym or trying new things when you don't really know what will work and what won't work. This book will help draw a path for your journey to better health. It's no brainer that you've heard the word' fasting' at one point in your life or another, regardless of culture, religion or race. Fasting has been observed in various forms throughout the centuries; many great philosophers like Plato also discuss it. It may be a central part of their religion or it may be performed as a religious activity preparatory training. This was also used as a way for getting rid of waste or contaminants that may have collected in the skin after a long period of time, cleaning people's minds and even removing excess body fat for weight loss.

Fasting's weight loss role is the main reason why in this day and age it has become so common. The worldwide increase in obesity is attributed to the fact that most people adopt traditional practice by eating low-fat food, not skipping meals and doing a lot of exercises. It is mostly based on opinions and is not motivated by concrete evidence and facts. The book will expose you to the magic of intermittent fasting, the fact-proven eating process.

Did you know that your body was designed to be fast, regardless of your size? Foodstuffs were difficult to come by this we're a product of drought and fantastic feasts; there wasn't really a middle ground. Intermittent fasting fits what our systems are used to, and the body likes it more than the three meals a day program. We feed for long periods of time on a daily basis but are constantly famished; this is an outcome made possible by electronic devices like televisions. Many are not happy with their bodies or the state in which their health is in. You can lose weight with the aid of intermittent fasting and also improve your health in the long term.

Most people have the wrong impression about fasting; they feel it's about lack of nutrition or starvation. Starving is a condition in which an individual does not have access to or wants food and eating it is not in their control. Where you are not in control of the situation or where your next food comes from is a complete and total mystery for you. Fasting is a choice and does not deprive you of food, unlike starving, which has absolutely no health benefits. The good thing about fasting is that it can function as it depends on why you do so. If it's done the right way, it can actually be done every day.

Chapter 1: What Is Intermittent Fasting?

In this chapter, we will talk about intermittent fasting and what it means to follow intermittent fasting. If you have been living under a rock, there's a high chance that you have no idea what intermittent fasting is or what it can do for you. What we will do is go through the basics of intermittent fasting so that you understand what intermittent fasting is and that you have a better understanding of it moving on. A quick disclaimer, this chapter might be boring too many people as the information is very remedial. However, this information to some might be new, so if you find this chapter boring, then you are free to skip it. However, if you're still iffy about intermittent fasting or that you have no idea on exactly what it does, then we recommend that you stick around. Time and time again, people have followed different types of fad diets, which may or may not work for them. Even if they do work for them, chances are they would give up very quickly and gain back the weight or the results that they achieved. The reason why they would give up and go back to the normal cell is that it is straightforward not to make it a habit or to make it a lifestyle.

The problem with modern-day and fad diets is that it is simply not sustainable in the long-term. If you want to lose weight and feel better by yourself for the rest of your life, then you need to pick something which is not only sustainable but can be adjusted into your lifestyle based on your needs. Moreover, you need something that gives you the freedom to eat and have whatever it is that you like in moderation so that you can enjoy life and be with your friends and family a lot more often. The truth is, many fad diets do not allow you to eat food, which is unhealthy. Don't get me wrong; eating unhealthy food all the time is not the best thing for your body anyways.

However, we recommend that you eat decent quality food often so that you see the benefits that you are looking for when it comes to losing fat or building muscle. However, eating decent food all the time can be a tedious task, which can lead to failure in the long-term, which is why having unhealthy food which tastes good here and there can lead to overall success in the long-term. With that being said, following fat diets play does not allow you to eat anything which is unhealthy. Most of the time, the fad diets put you in a position where you are insanely starving your body. Starving your body in the short-term might lead to weight loss, which might make you feel better, however starving yourself in the long-term can lead to many unwanted health fallbacks.

This is another reason why people who start following fad diets tend to give up so soon. This is where intermittent fasting comes in; the great thing about intermittent fasting is that many people don't even switch up what they are eating. What they do is eat cyclically. They would eat for certain hours of the day and would not eat for certain hours of the day. In essence, intermittent fasting is a cyclical way of eating. Now the most common way for people to follow intermittent fasting would be the 16/8 method. And this method you will be eating for 8 hours of the day, and you will be fasting for 16 hours of the day.

This is where you will not get any food to eat, and we'll have to survive on water or black coffee. You can have anything you want, which has no calories when you are fasting. Now there are tons of intermittent fasting methods which we will talk about later on in this book. However, the 16/8 method has been working very well for most people and can be added to their lifestyle. The great thing about this method would be that you don't have to worry about having certain hours to be more important than others when it comes to eating window and visa-versa. You will be the one picking out the times for your eating window and your fasting window. The most common times for fasting are 8 pm till 12 pm the next day, then eating from 12 pm to 8 pm, again this time could be whatever works for your schedule.

Another great thing about intermittent fasting would be that there are no restrictions on what you could be eating. For example, during the eating window, many people eat whatever they want within reason to achieve their goals. I have seen many

Fitness professionals eat food such as buttermilk biscuit, or even candy and dessert sometimes during the eating window, and still lose weight. We don't recommend you do that. However, this plan gives you the freedom to eat whatever you want while still seeing the results when it comes to losing fat and building muscle.

If you want to lose fat even more efficiently when intermittent fasting, we recommend that you eat a good, well-balanced diet slightly in a caloric deficit. This will allow you to not only lose fat but also to be certain that you're going to see results in the long-term when it comes to overall health and well-being. We also recommend that you accompany this with a fitness plan, make sure that you're working out in the gym if you want to lose fat and see the results that you have been hoping for. Another great thing about intermittent fasting, especially for people who are over the age of 50 years, is that it slows aging. One of the very best things, when it comes to intermittent fasting would be that it allows you to have very well-balanced aging and to make you look younger. These are thanks to two things, and the first one would be the increase in growth hormone. As you may know, intermittent fasting has shown to increase growth hormone production. This hormone is the youth of foundation, the reason why is because it will help you to recover quickly.

The benefits of growth hormone also include better skin and better bones, and you will also lose more fat and build more muscle. Another thing that intermittent fasting helps with would be the process known as autophagy. Autophagy is a process where your body gets rid of old/dead cells and replaces them with new cells.

This is the reason why you see the youth benefits, and also the reason why many people stay young for a very long time. These detoxifying cells would also mean getting rid of any diseased cells, which may include cancerous cells. Many people claim to get rid of their cancer very quickly by following intermittent fasting, and we can't back that up; however, it has been claimed by many cancer survivors. If you're someone looking to not only be better when it comes to Performance inside and outside the gym but also to look a lot younger in the long-term, then you have no reason why not to follow intermittent fasting. We will make it very easy for you when it comes to picking out the right plan and how to follow it appropriately.

Understand this, and intermittent fasting could be one of the easiest plans you could follow. And it all starts by reading this book. Do you have already taken the first step to seeing better results with your body and health, so make sure that you go all the way with it. Intermittent fasting is like eating in increments. As we told you, it is a cyclical way of eating food, which allows you to consume all the calories you need in a certain hour of the day. While certain of the day, you will be fasting and not eating anything at all. Once you start following intermittent fasting, you will be surprised how much time we spend on eating food. We spend a lot of time, more specifically waste a lot of time eating food. If you're someone who is looking to see success with their business or their work environment, then you will gain from that time and see the results that you have been hoping for. Intermittent fasting truly is a win-win situation. It makes you feel younger, and it gets rid of any bad cells in your body while increasing all the good hormones. Think of it this way, and there are many people who follow intermittent fasting without even knowing it. Many religions recommend that you fast for 30 days, or however long. This goes to show intermittent fasting has been in practice for a very long time, and good reason, it simply works.

Now, if you are someone who can't fast every day for the rest of your life, don't worry as you will have at least one day in the week or you can eat throughout the whole day. We recommend that you do that as it will allow you to be more motivated in the long-term, which is what intermittent fasting is all about is creating a lifestyle. If you are tired of following diets that yield you some results, but they aren't sustainable in the long-term, then chances are intermittent fasting is going to be your savior.

Make sure that you pick the plan that fits your needs and your goals. We will talk about all the intermittent fasting methods later on in this book. However, once you understand the benefits and the reasons why you need to be following intermittent fasting, then it will be straightforward for you to follow it in the long-term. The main thing that differentiates intermittent fasting to any other fad diet is that they're health benefits to intermittent fasting and not just aesthetic benefits. Meaning, God guides give you a set of promises which may or may not be delivered. However, intermittent fasting has shown time and time again to deliver aesthetic benefits, and on top of that, help you get rid of many diseases that will help you stay healthy for a very long time.

Intermittent fasting is also one of the best plans to follow up for someone who's over the age of 50. The reasons why we told you is because it helps you to say younger and to enjoy life a lot more when you're 50 the main thing you want to do is enjoy the life, if you want to enjoy life then you need to be in a healthy State of Mind and Body. Intermittent fasting gives you all of that, and on top of that, it helps you to say a lot younger for a very long time. If you don't believe me, then look at your celebrities, many celebrities who are in their 50s tend to follow intermittent fasting and for an excellent reason. It is because it helps them to stay younger and to think a lot better and quickly.

Finally, intermittent fasting helps you to save a lot more time because you will not be thinking about eating for a certain amount of time, which will allow you to spend that time working on your craft. With that being said, we now conclude this chapter. The main take-home message from this chapter would be that intermittent fasting can be used for numerous reasons, if you are someone looking to gain muscle or lose fat or you want to be younger for a long time. Also, intermittent fasting is something that should be considered more of a lifestyle than something which is to be done once every two months. Now, if you are serious about changing your life, and about starting living healthier than intermittent fasting is the answer for you.

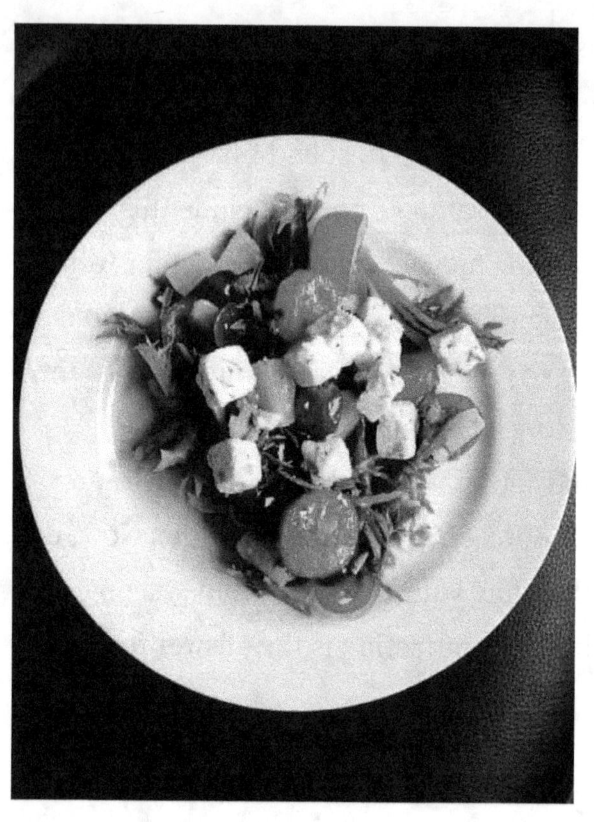

Chapter 2: How Intermittent Fasting Works

Our body can handle extended periods of not eating. Human bodies have the natural ability to transition between the hunger state and the full state. When we don't eat for a long period of time, the processes going inside our body change. When we eat our body starts to work on digesting it and storing the energy received through the meal. When we are hungry, our body starts to take energy from those stored fats.

When we are fasted for a specific period of time, our blood sugar and insulin levels face a reduction in their levels. It is normal because it pushes our body to thrive from existing resources present inside our bodies. Researches have shown that fasting helps to protect against diseases like heart diseases, diabetes, cancer and Alzheimer's disease. Therefore, when in a fasted state, you shouldn't worry that you shouldn't worry that it will affect your health.

In order to understand how intermittent fasting works, two states have to be understood first. The two states are – the fed state and the fasted state. By understanding these states, we get to know that how our bodies keep functioning well regardless of the fact that our stomachs are empty or full.

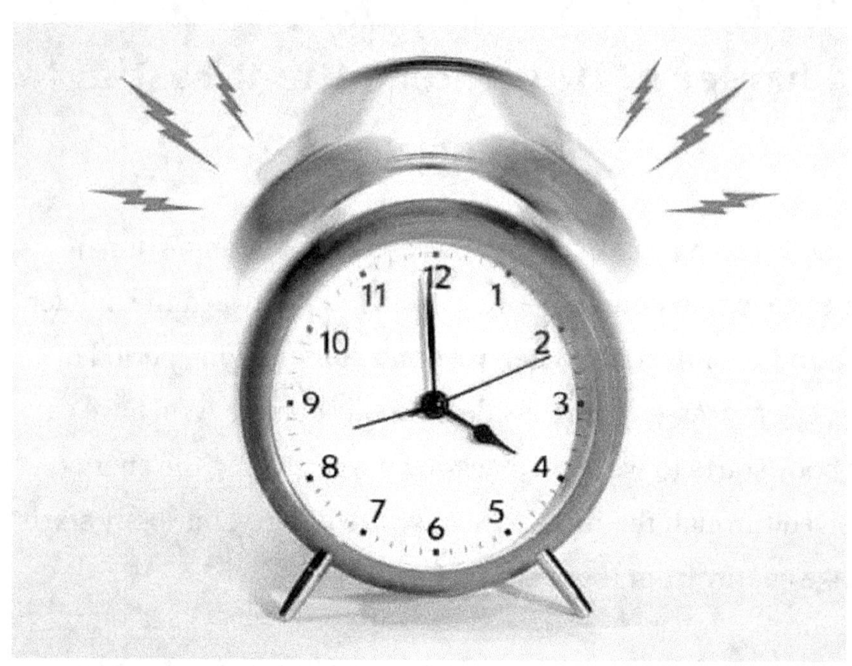

Two IF States: Fed vs. Fasted

In the Fed state, the body is undergoing process of digesting and absorbing food. The state begins when you start eating and can last from three to five hours after that. In fed state, your body shows elevated levels of insulin, and this acts as a signal for your body to store the excess amounts of calories. This storage takes place in the fat cells. During the time with high insulin levels, the process of fat burning comes to a stop and the body shifts towards burning glucose from your last meal instead.

Then a state called post-absorptive state comes, which lasts about 8 to 12 hours after the last meal. After that the body enters the Fasted state. In the Fasted state; body is not processing any meal and the levels of insulin are low. This induces a mobilization of stored body fat presiding inside the body in the fat cells and starts to burn these fats for providing energy to the body. In this state, the body can burn the fat that was first inaccessible to it during the fed state.

Staying hungry for a specific duration of time helps you with hundreds of things. When you eat a meal, your body is under 'fed state' and is just processing the meal you just ate. After a few hours pass and the food is completely digested, it goes into a mid-stage where you don't feel hungry but you haven't eaten anything else yet. You can call this an intermediate state. After 8 to 12 hours from your last meal, a state comes called 'fasted state' when you feel hungry and you are under a fast. In this state, your body needs to re-gain the fuel to work but it doesn't find any energy being provided to it. So, it starts to look for energy sources inside the body. It starts to go towards the fat cells where fats from your previous meals have been stored. The body is designed to store some amount of fat from every meal in order to regain energy at the time when it is needed. Thus, because of low insulin levels now the body has entered into a fat-burning state and it starts to burn the fats present inside the body. This is beneficial in hundreds of ways. It will not only get rid of the excess fat from you, but will also get rid of any toxins present inside a body.

The toxins can be anything harmful present in your body. It can be dysfunctional cell or a cell that is damaged and is not performing well. Removal of such cells is very necessary when we talk about maintaining health. So, you have to be under the 'fasted state' so that your body can initialize the burn-off state. Intermittent fasting provides you a convenient way to enter into the fasted state and get rid of all excess fats, calories and damaged cells. Many health-practitioners and doctors advise their patients to start fasting for this purpose. They believe that health will improve if they fast because of this quality of intermittent fasting.

Chapter 3: Is Intermittent Fasting Good for Women?

Female participants in studies across the globe and those reporting their personal results on social media or within fitness communities report many of the same negative effects felt by men throughout the course of adjusting to a new Intermittent Fasting plan. Some of these side effects include:

•Initial hunger pangs and dehydration

•Difficulty concentrating or gaining focus throughout the day

•Headaches, muscle weakness, initial loss in muscle tone

There are some effects that women have experienced and should be watched out for, especially those with a history of trouble or concerns with their menstrual cycles. One such negative effect reported is infertility after long periods of time on an Intermittent Fasting plan. This tends to happen more in women who see a dramatic loss in body fat, especially in the first few weeks (or during the adjustment time).

•In most women, this is nothing to be permanently concerned about as typically periods return to normal and fertility increases in the weeks after stopping an Intermittent Fasting plan, particularly for weight loss reasons

•Most wellness experts and medical professionals recommend that women who may be pregnant, are pregnant or are hoping to become pregnant in the near future avoid starting or cease their Intermittent Fasting plan in order to ensure they are in peak condition for childbearing or do not minimize their chances of conceiving

However, for those worried about starting an Intermittent Fasting routine, it is important to point out that even though fasting is still being studied around the world for its long-term benefits and risks on nearly anyone who could ever be interested in trying it (different ages, genders, races, cultural diets, health histories), health and wellness experts all over have written and spoken about its safety, its benefits and its promising progress for men and women alike. It all comes down to being prepared; having all the right information and making a plan that will work and can be stuck with for the long run.

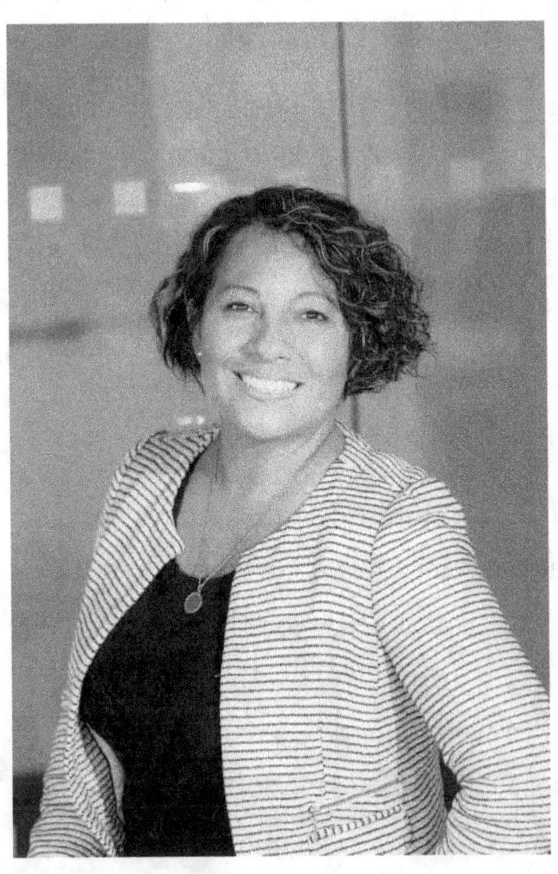

Advantages of Intermittent Fasting

Intermittent fasting has incredible benefits not only to women's body and brain but also to men's. The following are a few of the benefits linked to intermittent starvation:

Altering the functioning of body cells and hormones: Intermittent fasting practiced for a while brings several alterations in your body. For your body to make more fats accessible, it tends to initiate significant cell repair processes and also changes the levels of hormones in your body. The levels of insulin in your body drop facilitating the breakdown of fats. Growth hormones also increase as the blood levels in them increase a factor that facilitates muscle gaining. The body induces processes such as cellular repairing and removal of any waste materials from the cells.

Lose of weight and belly calories: Intermittent fasting is done to lose weight as you only take in a few meals. Intermittent fasting enhances your metabolic rate, which helps your body burn excess fats such as the belly fats. Studies show that intermittent fasting leads to a 3-8 percent weight loss if done for around three to twenty-four weeks. Observation shows that within this fasting duration, four to seven percent of people lost their belly fats, one of the toxic fats in a human's body responsible for various illnesses.

Reduces the resistance of insulin: Intermittent fasting reduces the insulin levels in your body, that in turn lowers risks of Type 2 Diabetes, which has been a common illness. The common characteristics of diabetes include high levels of blood sugar in the situation of insulin battle. Thus, intermittent fasting helps in lowering the levels of insulin, which helps in preventing this illness. It also helps protect any possible damages that can affect your kidneys.

Reduction of oxidative constant worry and body inflammation: Intermittent fasting helps reduce stress, which is one of the riskiest ways of fast aging as well as other chronic illnesses. Free radicals are the molecules responsible for reacting with molecules such as DNA and proteins and destroy them. Intermittent fasting, therefore, helps fight body inflammation and destroy any molecules responsible for constant worries.

Heart health: Intermittent fasting is beneficial for your heart's health and prevents you against any heart diseases. Since it regulates sugar levels in your body, intermittent fasting prevents you from high blood pressure, and inflammatory markers, and cholesterol levels hence maintaining the heart health.

Induction of cellular restoration procedures: When you fast, your body initiates the cell's 'waste elimination' procedures that are known as autophagy. Body cells break down and metabolize the dysfunctional proteins that accumulate inside the body cells. Increased waste elimination prevents your body against other illnesses such as Alzheimer's disease, one of the common neurodegenerative disorders with no cure.

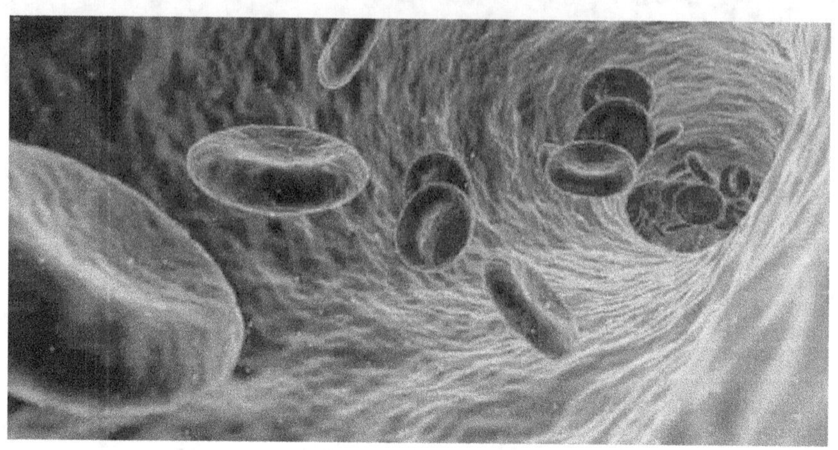

Prevention against cancer: After your body eliminates any dysfunctional cells that accumulate over time, your body becomes free from any cancer risks. The uncontrolled development of cells is one of the common characteristics of cancer, and therefore, intermittent fasting facilitates your body's metabolic rate, which helps reduce any possible risks of cancer. Intermittent fasting also reduces several impacts of chemotherapy.

Brain health: Since intermittent fasting is better for your body, then it is best for your brain. Reduction of oxidative stress and various worries is advantageous for your brain fitness. Recurrent fasting increases the development of new nerves, which improves the functioning of your brain. It also helps in increasing brain hormone levels known as the Brain-derived neurotrophic factors, which helps fight depression and any other brain-related illnesses. Intermittent fasting also helps fight brain damages caused by stroke.

Extending lifespan: Intermittent fasting can help you live longer due to its ability to control metabolism rates, regulating blood sugar levels, and eliminating any dysfunctional cells within your body.

Disadvantages of Intermittent Fasting

Unfortunately, intermittent fasting has cons too, especially to the females. Studies show that before trying intermittent fasting, you should always contact your physician. The following are the disadvantages associated with intermittent fasting:

It is not risk-free: Intermittent fasting is not advisable to people who are at higher health risks such as those over sixty-five years. People under medical conditions, high fat needs, the diabetic, the underweight, the underage, pregnant, and those breastfeeding cannot undertake intermittent fasting.

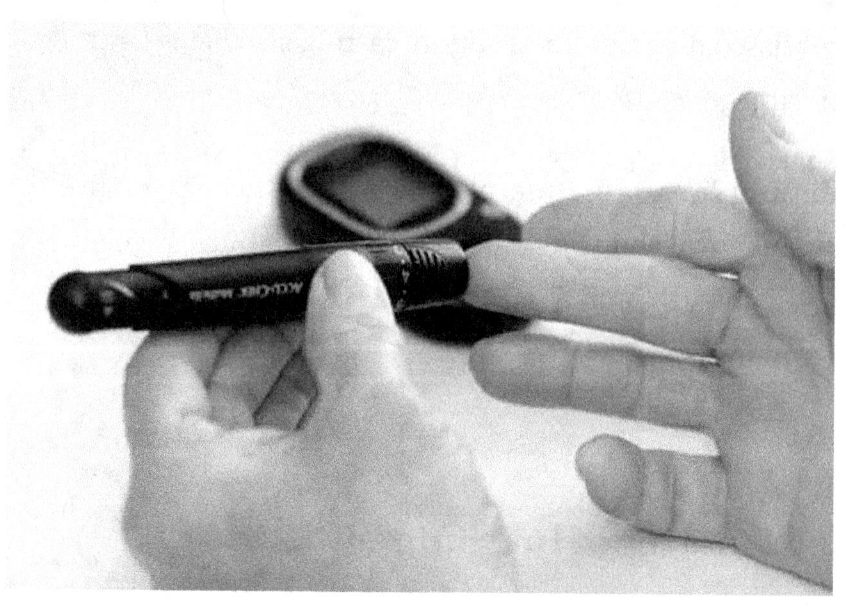

You will be hungry: During intermittent fasting, you might have grumbling stomach, especially if you have correctly been observing the correct dietary plans. You should avoid looking at, smelling, or even thinking about food while fasting since these triggers the releasing o gastric acids in your stomach, which then makes you hungry. Engage in some other activities but if you wish to fill your water, drink herbal tea or other drinks free from calories. You may note increased food intake in the non-eating days where you are not limited to any calorie intakes. Intermittent fasting triggers binge food consumption. There could also be cases of cravings, especially after increased levels of cortisol hormone.

Dehydration: Lack of eating may make you forget to take water. You might fail to take note of the thirst cues when fasting.

Fatigue: Intermittent fasting makes you feel tired, especially if you are trying it for the first time. Your body tends to run short of energy and disrupts your sleep patterns, and this comes along with a feeling of being tired.

Irritability: Since intermittent fasting helps in mood regulation, it can as well regulate your appetite. It leads to being depressed and upset.

Intermittent fasting long-term consequences are not known: Since no one knows whether after losing weight, you will maintain the same for some years, studies claim that no relevant evidence to support the extent of intermittent fasting. You are therefore always advised to talk to your doctor for sound advice on how you should practice intermittent fasting.

There are precautions that you should undertake when practicing intermittent fasting. Fasting has been there since time immemorial, and in some religions, it is considered as a holy practice. Whatever way, you may start practicing intermittent fasting; you should follow its essential tips to avoid any inconveniences.

Therefore, you should:

Ensure that your body is fit for fasting. It is by making sure that you are not pregnant, not under any medication, no health complications, not underage, or even diabetic. If you cannot fast, then you can always change to cleaner eating habits such as eating natural foods and eliminate any sugar, rich, or fatty foods from your diet.

Before starting intermittent fasting, you should always try and consult your doctor. Your doctor will give updates about your health concerns and advise whether the step is necessary or not.

Try and make intermittent fasting fit into your lifestyle.
You should never fast during the times you are stressed or under
excess exertion. It is advisable if you are a newbie in
intermittent fasting to try the 5:2 way of fasting whereby you can
fast on the first day of the week, then on Thursdays so that you
can prepare to take your favorite meals over the weekend.

Before you start intermittent fasting, do not gorge yourself with
a 'last supper' but you should instead take healthy meals, lean
proteins, and vegetables. Fruits have natural sugar, and
including them in your meal could mean a lot. A little amount of
starch could make the meal complete, as well. A meal that has
all these nutrients will make your body survive the fasting
period.

**Prepare your household, body, and thoughts before
starting intermittent fasting.** It means that you should have
enough rest and get prepared emotionally. Think about your aim
and how to achieve it. Make sure that you hide or keep out of
reach any foods that could tempt you during your fasting
period.

Stop pretending to be a hero, even when your body is weak. Do
not push your body too hard in the name of fasting. There are
some of the symptoms that should be of great concern during
your fasting time. You should take note of heart shudders, lightheadedness, and general feebleness. It requires the use of

common sense because you cannot force your body to do what it cannot.

Do not engage in tough exercises; do light ones. Engage in massages as they help have even blood flow in the body parts full of calories, thus reducing cortisol. Do not burn the muscles for energy while fasting.

Always take your vitamins depending on the method of fasting you choose. That acts as a supplement, especially if in liquid form as it eases the process of digestion. They help compensate the vitamins lost while fasting.

Never forget to take a lot of water every fasting day. Your urine should alert you if it is not light in color. If not so, drink desirable amounts of water for proper hydration.

Since you are fasting, it is an obstacle to associating with your friends who are having fun; eating chocolates and drinking wine since you will get tempted to take some. You can indulge in other ways of having fun with your friends. You can pay a visit to the nearest mall, window-shop new clothes or electronics. Avoid grocery stores and any dinner dates. Clear any mouth-watering photos from your gallery.

Avoid getting stressed since stress increases the levels of cortisol, which is responsible for fat storage and muscle breakdown. You can practice yoga, meditating, or having deep breaths. Your body needs enough energy to last you during the fasting period, and so these exercises should be light and not vigorous.

To avoid freaking out, you can always invite your friends to accompany you in doing intermittent fasting. The idea of creating your fasting thread or checking online for any other people doing intermittent fasting can help you master your progress. That is the time that you should focus on mentally cleaning your closet and reflecting on what you are doing.

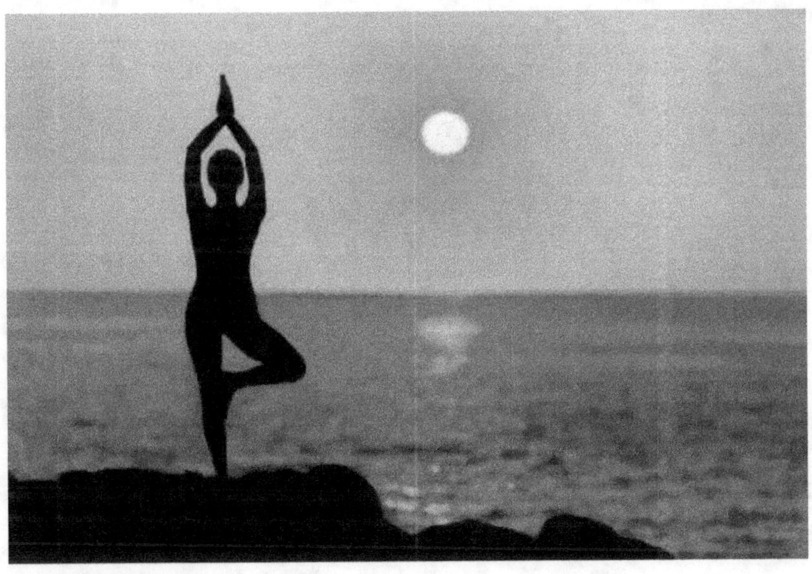

Avoid 'Victory Binging.' Many people indulge themselves after the fasting period. You should take in a healthy meal and avoid foods that cannot get digested easily. You should take in foods rich in fiber and if you are alcoholic, remember to take care when resuming.

Chapter 4: The Differences between the Young vs Older Woman

While the greatest concerns about intermittent fasting's effects on women often center on potential problems with reproduction and fertility, some women simply don't have to worry about that anymore. For mature and menopausal women, intermittent fasting poses a different instance and option entirely.

This chapter will be dedicated to the experiences of these women. It will discuss what happens when women age, how their needs change, and how nutrition is affected. Furthermore, it will discuss how intermittent fasting affects both mature and menopausal women before giving suggestions of how to approach IF for each type of woman.

Next, we will walk through some anti-aging foods, tips, and exercises to lose that weight, and then we'll end with the best intermittent fasting method for you at this time. By the time this chapter ends, you should feel confident (as a mature or menopausal woman) that you can approach intermittent fasting safely and productively, and you should have a solid plan in mind regarding how you'll go about that when you're ready.

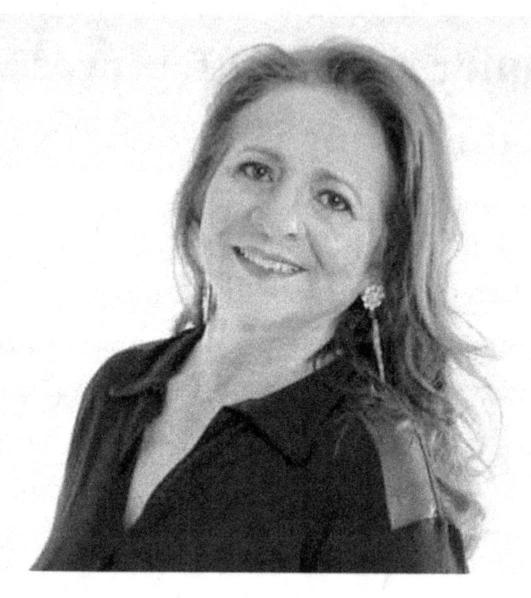

Differences Between the Young vs. Older Woman

At the most basic level, it must be said that there are detailed bodily differences between young women and older women. Many of these bodily differences become obvious with the outward, physical effects of aging, but a lot of them also happen on the inside, away from what our eyes can see.

When women age, enter and exit menopause, and become fully mature, their bodies change, reflecting different nutritional needs for the next 30+ years. During menopause, in particular, certain foods help with the urges, hot flashes, and more, but the period of intense transition is more of a gateway into a completely altered future (mentally, bodily, nutritionally, and more).

Women of this age experience slowed metabolism (to their great frustrations) as well as lowered hormone production. For weight and mood, therefore, menopause and maturation are equal disasters. Your body will go completely "out of whack," compared to how it used to function. You'll likely put on weight despite the dietary choices you make, and you may feel there's no relief in sight. Don't be fooled, however! Things may have changed for you, but they won't be stagnant changes.

Essentially, women at the stage of menopause and beyond need to absorb less energy overall from their food, yet they need more protein to deal with the effects of aging. Vitamins B12 & D, calcium, and zinc will need to be boosted, while iron becomes less important for the aging female body. Vitamins C, E, A, & beta-carotene need to be increased too in order to fight off cancer, infection, disease, and more.

As the woman ages and matures even further, more things will change; mainly, she cannot bypass taking these important supplements any longer. In older and more mature women, the body's abilities to recognize hunger and thirst become muted, and dehydration poses a greater threat. Fewer calories are required for the older and more mature woman too, but she still needs to get as many nutrients as (if not more than!) the young woman does.

It seems that a younger woman can eat (relatively) what she wants and not worry about taking vitamins or supplements, but it is undeniable that the older woman will need this nutritional help to *ensure* longevity. Basically, health needs become more pressing for women at this age, as their bodies are less flexible and resistant to problems that may arise.

How IF Affects Women at this Age and How to Approach It

Because health, diet, reproductivity, and nutritional needs are all altered for mature and menopausal women, their relationships with intermittent fasting can be very different from young women's. For instance, while young women ought to be careful about how intermittent fasting can affect their fertility levels, older women can practice intermittent fasting freely without these concerns. Therefore, more mature women can apply the weight-loss techniques of intermittent fasting to their lives (and waistlines) without worry of what negative side-effects might arise in the future.

For menopausal women, however, the situation is a little bit different than it is for fully mature women. People going through menopause have to deal with daily hormone fluctuations that cause hot and cold flashes, sleeplessness, anxiety, irregular periods, and more. At the beginning of this process, intermittent fasting *will not* necessarily help, and it could even make your situation more stressful.

For women in this situation who are actively going through menopause, you must remember that your body is extremely sensitive to changes right now. If you do find that intermittent fasting helps and that short periods of fast are effective, you *must* also make sure to increase the intensity of your fast as gradually as possible so your body can adjust without creating horrible hormonal repercussions for yourself and everyone around you.

For the fully mature woman, intermittent fasting will not make you as cranky, moody, irregular in the period, or otherwise because those hormones won't be affecting you at all anymore, or at least, hardly at all. Your dietary and eating schedule choices become more liberated from the effects they used to have on your hormonal health as the years go by. Therefore, if you're seeking weight loss, better energy, a physiological jolt back to health, or what have you, try out IF without concern and see what happens. For these types of women, intermittent fasting is set to provide hope through eased depression, the lessened likelihood of cancer (or its recurrence), promised weight loss, and more.

Anti-Aging Foods

Avocado is high in omega-3s, which help your immune system as well as your body as a whole fight inflammation.

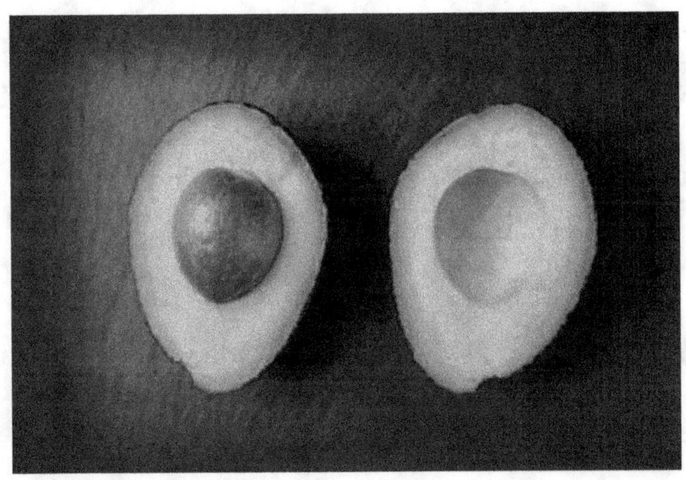

Beans & Lentils are great sources of protein and fiber, particularly for older women.

Blueberries are high in vitamin C and antioxidants that help protect the skin from pollutants, sun exposure, aging stress, and more.

Broccoli, Cauliflower, & Brussel Sprouts are all relatively high in lutein which keeps your brain healthy and sharp!

Carrots are also rich in vitamin A as well as beta-carotene which helps your vision later in life.

Cilantro might taste like soap to some, but it helps remove metals from your body that shouldn't be there. It's a great detoxifier for women of any age.

Cooked Tomatoes have a powerful antioxidant present that helps the skin heal from the damage of any kind.

Dark Chocolate is packed with flavanols (which aid in the appearance of the skin and protect against the damage of the sun).

Edamame aids in bone health, cardiovascular healing, and ease into lowered estrogen levels with menopause.

Fortified Plant-Based Milk is a great non-dairy alternative to the "healing" animal milk you may know and love. They provide bone-supportive minerals and nutrients like calcium and vitamin D (as long as they're fortified!) without adding in the problematic nature of dairy to your healthy drink.

Ghee is a special form of clarified butter that is packed with healthy fats for skin health and detoxification.

Green Tea de-stresses the body and mind and blocks DNA from damage in many forms.

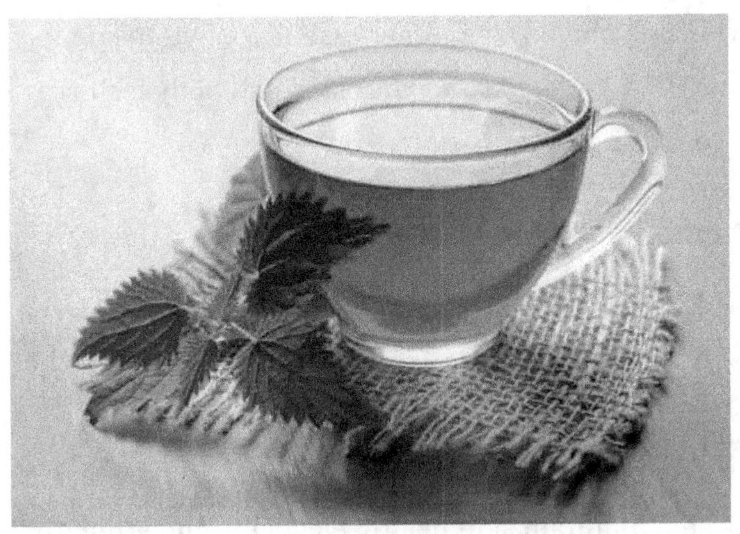

Manuka Honey is a special type of honey that's a powerful natural remedy for immune boost and skin health.

Mushrooms are high in vitamin D, which is so important for women of all ages.

Nuts are great at lowering cholesterol and fighting inflammation. They're also packed with fiber, protein, and micronutrients.

Oatmeal provides carbohydrates that encourage the release of serotonin, which keeps you feeling good.

Olives provide polyphenols and other essential phytonutrients that keep your DNA protected and your skin and body feeling and looking young.

Oranges, Lemons, & Limes, when juiced, provide the greatest source of healthy vitamin C you can imagine.

Papaya has many antioxidants, vitamins, and minerals that keep the skin elastic with fewer wrinkle lines.

Pineapples help maintain skin health, elasticity, and strength as you age.

Pomegranate Seeds are also high in antioxidants, and they're great at fighting free radical molecules that encourage the effects of aging on the body.

Red & Orange Bell Peppers have antioxidants and high vitamin C to help the skin retain its healthy shine while protecting it against pollutants and toxins.

Red Wine, when drunk in moderation, is a powerful tool to keep your heart healthy, lower cholesterol, and maintain muscle mass.

Saffron has anti-tumor, antioxidant, and other highly nutritious effects for the body.

Sesame Seeds will help you feel good through their high levels of calcium, magnesium, fiber, phosphorous, and iron.

Spinach & Other Leafy Greens work to protect the skin from sun damage while providing beta-carotene and lutein to solidify that effect.

Sweet Potato has more vitamin A than regular potatoes, which keeps your skin fresh and young-looking without lines and wrinkles.

Turmeric is great for the skin and for keeping the organs working in tip-top shape. The pigment curcumin also helps to heal DNA and prevent degenerative diseases.

Watercress is a happily hydrating green that's high in phosphorous, manganese, calcium, potassium, vitamins A, C, K, B1, and B2.

Watermelon works like a natural sun blocker when eaten and provides a great source of water to keep you hydrated.

Yogurt helps your cells stay young and is often probiotic, which is great for healthy gut flora and mood stabilization.

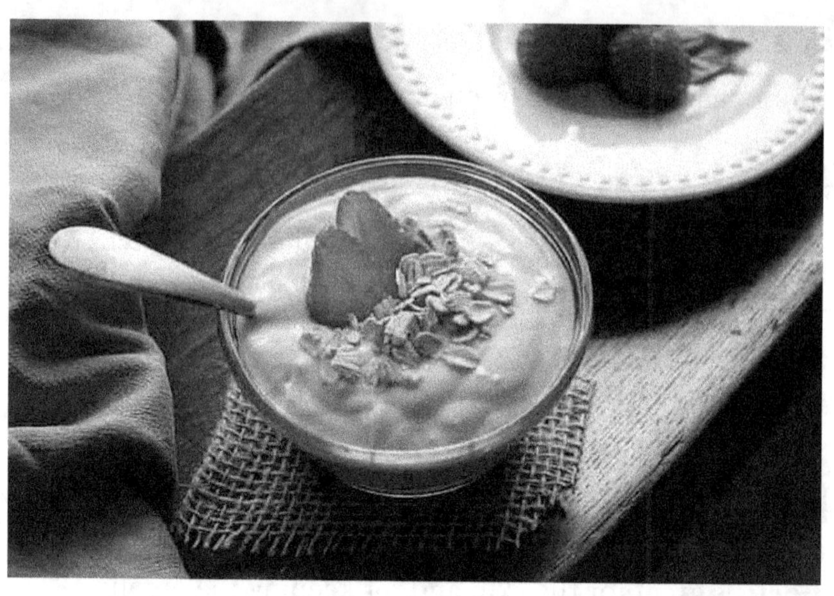

Tips and Exercises to Lose Belly Fat and Kickstart your Metabolism

If you're eager to lose that belly fat associated with menopause and give your metabolism a kick-start to the face, you're definitely in the right place! Whether or not you choose to incorporate intermittent fasting into your life, there are still several things you can do to make sure these goals are achieved exactly as you want them to be.

The two biggest tips for losing this belly fat are (1) to switch your diet to something that triggers fat loss and fat burning and (2) to start a new exercise regimen. While the intermittent fasting plan is not technically a diet, this switch in when you eat might be exactly what you need. If not, however, a few true diets you can try are The Low-Carb Diet, whereby you reduce the number of carbs you take in each day; The Mediterranean Diet, which is essentially vegetarian and plant-based aside from the occasional red meat and a few other switches; the Vegetarian Diet, which is shown to be particularly effective at helping overweight post-menopausal women lose the fat they desire; and then the more intense Vegan Diet, which boasts the same effects as The Vegetarian Diet, just with more conclusive, less age-restrictive results.

Altering your diet is just one step, however. You also have to be exercising enough to burn the fat that's present. Given your age, your ability, and any other circumstances, you'll want to find a mode of exercise that's not too demanding or stressful. Somethings that could work for you are Resistance Training with low weights and bands, Aerobic Cardio, Aerobic Exercise otherwise, and Low-Demand Strength Training. Daily walks are also incredibly helpful for women in your situation to be able to reach their weight loss goals. If you can manage it, a combination of Aerobic and Resistance Exercises is ideal.

Best (IF) Methods for Health and Weight Loss at this Age

For the menopausal woman, the best method to start with would be something low-stress and gradual. The crescendo method sure is gradual, but it may be a little too intense for the menopausal woman to use as a beginner. If you do start with a crescendo, try two days a week at 12:12 or 14:10 at the toughest. If that feels okay, that's great, but you still should probably not make things any more forceful.

Instead of trying the crescendo method whatsoever, I would suggest the woman in this situation try spontaneous skip method first to see how things feel. If she's too moody, frustrated, hot-flashy, and upset with just this adjustment, I suggest she wait a few months until trying intermittent fasting again. If this phase goes well, she can up the ante and try 12:12 method, then 14:10 and 16:8 when she's ready. I doubt the menopausal woman would want to venture beyond these first four starting methods, however, given the bodily situation she's working through.

On the flip side, **for the fully mature, post-menopausal woman**, any method would be fine to start with. If the woman is unsure about starting off with day-by-day fierceness in her IF experience, she can try working with 12:12 method, working up to 14:10 method, and 16:8 if things feel okay. Even crescendo method would work well for the woman in this situation because she could determine how strict the "day-by-day" aspect was and make the schedule work in her favor. Any woman in this case likely won't *want* to start with the most rigorous intermittent fast, so these hourly-based ones offer a smoother initial transition.

If the woman in this situation has worked with intermittent fasting before, she is free to choose whichever method she prefers. If the mature woman has established a career for herself later in life and lives full days with evenings free, she is invited to try the warrior method. As long as she's taking supplements and drinking enough liquids, even this strenuous, appropriately-named diet can even be tackled by the oldest of women among us!

Chapter 5: How Intermittent Fasting Affects Women at this Age and How to Approach It

There are plenty of diets out there, all promising you the impossible. Incredible weight loss, with no mention of any side effects. You are probably fed up with the "lose x pounds in 30 days, guaranteed" approach. Many of these diets are not backed up by science, or in other words, there is not any scientific research to prove these diets actually deliver what they promise. They focus only on the weight loss process, suggesting meal plans that are extremely radical in some cases.

Diets mean nutrient deprivation in most cases, but they are plenty of cases when these diets have harmful effects on your health. Unlike other diets, focused on the weight loss process in an incredibly short amount of time, intermittent fasting is focusing more on your health, as nutritionists believe that health should be the most important factor, and only a healthy body can have a long and sustainable weight loss process. Unlike the other diets, which have a "hit and run" approach, IF is something for the long run and should be regarded as a way of life, not like a meal plan to be implemented for a few weeks. By checking out the benefits below, you can better understand why this process is so beneficial for your body.

The main benefits of intermittent fasting can be summarized in 8 points:

•eliminates precancerous and cancerous cells

•shifts easily into nutritional ketosis

•reduces the fat tissue

•enhances the gene expression for health span and longevity

•induces autophagy and the apoptotic cellular repair or cleaning

•improves your insulin sensitivity

•reduces inflammation and oxidative stress

•increases neuroprotection and cognitive effects

To expand on the benefits of this practice, intermittent fasting can have positive impacts over the fat loss process, disease prevention, anti-aging, therapeutic benefits (psychological, spiritual and physical), mental performance, physical fitness (improved metabolism, wind, and endurance, the great effect over bodybuilding).

Intermittent Fasting for the Weight Loss Process

As you restrain yourself from eating, the body will no longer have available glucose to use in order to produce energy. Therefore, it will use ketones to break the fat tissue open and release the energy stored in there. This is how the body will burn your existing fat in order to generate energy. When it comes to diets, they are not designed for the long run, and as soon as you break the diet, you will start gaining weight again. Intermittent fasting is something that you can try for a lifetime because it is easy to stick to it, and it doesn't involve any special meal plan. So, you can still eat your favorite foods, as long as you schedule your meals, allowing a smaller eating window and a longer fasting period. IF induces ketosis and eventually autophagy, which will definitely mean reducing the fat reserves.

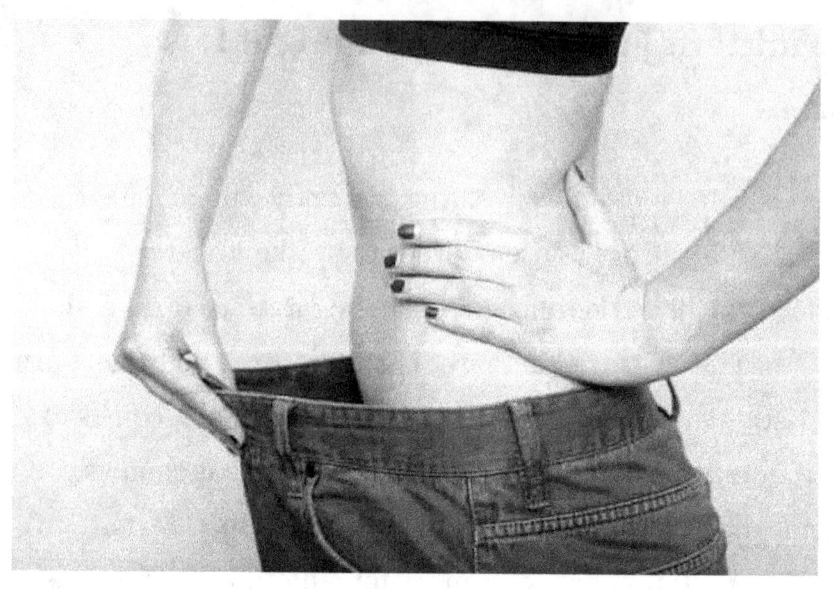

Intermittent Fasting for Preventing Diseases

What if you found out that intermittent fasting is, in fact, a cure for several different diseases and medical conditions? You would definitely become more interested in this process. There are a few studies that show the beneficial effects IF has on your health. A study published in the World Journal of Diabetes has shown that patients with type 2 diabetes on short-term daily intermittent fasting experience a lower body weight, but also a better variability of post-meal glucose.

Other benefits this diet has are:

•enhances the markers of stress resistance

•reduces the blood pressure and inflammation

•better lipid levels and glucose circulation, which may lead to a lower risk of cardiovascular disease, neurological diseases like Parkinson's and Alzheimer's, and also cancer

Intermittent Fasting for the Anti-Aging Process

The modern-day lifestyle includes too much stress and is too sedentary. Whether we like it or not, these factors have a great contribution to the aging process. You are probably wondering what intermittent fasting can do the slow down this process, as we all know that it can't be stopped. IF is not "the fountain of youth" and it will not grant you immortality, but it can still lower the blood pressure and reduce oxidative damage, enhance your insulin sensitivity and reduce your fat mass. Coincidence or not, all of these are factors are known to improve your health and longevity. Intermittent fasting is one of the triggering factors of autophagy, a process known for destroying and replacing old cell parts with new ones, at any level within your body. Such a process can slow down the aging process.

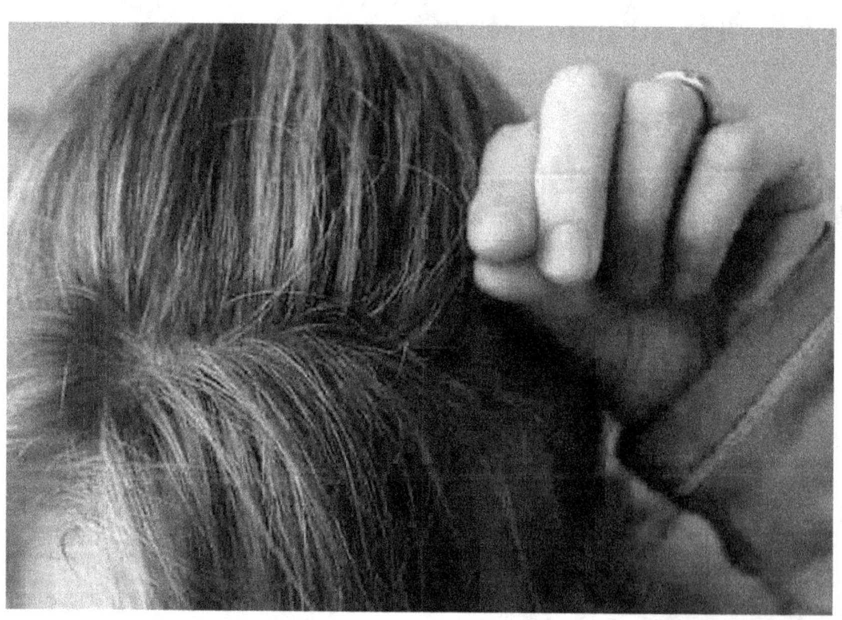

Intermittent Fasting Practiced for Therapeutic Benefits

When it comes to therapeutic benefits, the most important ones are physical, spiritual and psychological. In terms of physical benefits, intermittent fasting is a powerful cure for diabetes, but it can also prove to be very useful for reducing seizure-related brain damage and seizures themselves, but also for improving the symptoms of arthritis. This practice also has a spiritual value, as it's widely practiced for religious purposes across the globe. Although fasting is regarded as penance by some practitioners, it's also a practice for purifying your body and soul (according to the religious approach).

Intermittent fasting is also about exercising control and will, over your body and your feelings. Achieving absolute control over your power and mind is a very powerful psychological benefit. You can ignore hunger, restrain yourself from eating for a certain period of time. In other words, IF is also associated with mind training and can also improve your self-esteem. A successful intermittent fasting regime can have very powerful effects from a psychological point of view. A study has shown that women practicing IF had amazing results in terms of senses of control, reward, pride, and achievement.

Intermittent Fasting for Better Mental Performance

IF also enhances the cognitive function and also is very useful when it comes to boosting your brain power. There are several factors of intermittent fasting which can support this claim. First of all, it boosts the level of brain-derived neurotrophic factor (also known as BDNF), which is a protein in your brain that can interact with the parts of your brain responsible for controlling cognitive and memory functions as well as learning. BDNF can even protect and stimulate the growth of new brain cells. Through IF, you will enter the ketogenic state, during which your body turn fat into energy, by using ketones. Ketones can also feed your brain, and therefore improve your mental acuity, productivity, and energy.

Intermittent Fasting for an Improved Physical Fitness

This process influences not only your brain but also your digestive system. By setting a small feeding window and a larger fasting period, you will encourage the proper digestion of food. This leads to a proportional and healthy daily intake of food and calories. The more you get used to this process, the less you will experience hunger. If you are worried about slowing your metabolism, think again! IF enhances your metabolism, it makes metabolism more flexible, as the body has now the capability to run on glucose or fats for energy, in a very effective way. In other words, intermittent fasting leads to better metabolism.

Oxygen use during exercise is a crucial part of the success of your training. You simply can't have performance without adjusting your breathing habits during workouts. VO2 max represents the maximum amount of oxygen your body can use per minute or per kilogram of body weight. In popular terms, VO2 max is also referred to as "wind". The more oxygen you use, the better you will be able to perform. Top athletes can have twice the VO2 level of those without any training. A study focused on the VO2 levels of a fasted group (they just skipped breakfast) and a non-fasted group (they had breakfast an hour before). For both groups, the VO2 level was at 3.5 L/min at the beginning, and after the study, the level showed a significant increase of "wind" for the fasting group (9.7%), compared to just 2.5% increase in the case of those with breakfast.

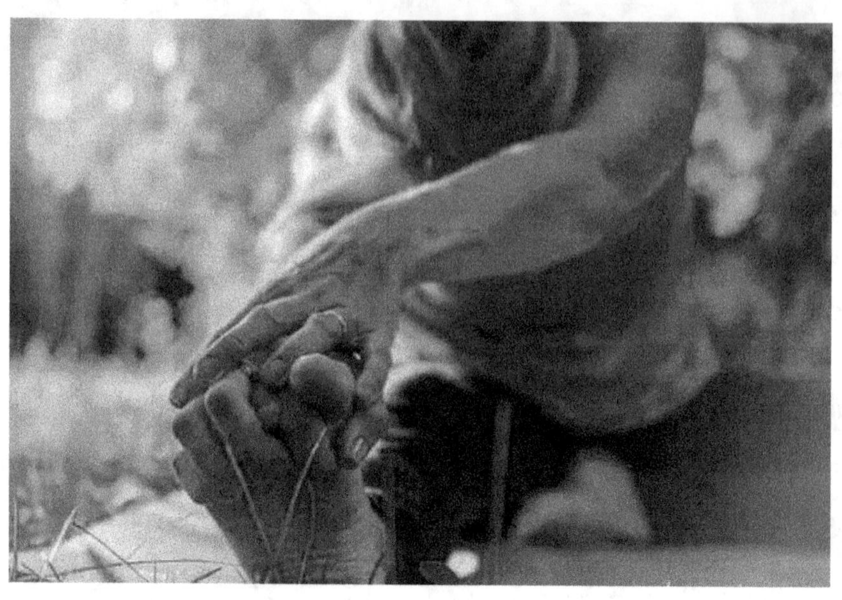

Intermittent Fasting for Bodybuilding

Having a narrow feeding window automatically mean fewer meals, so you can concentrate the daily calorie intake into just 1-2 consistent meals. Bodybuilders find this approach a lot more pleasing than having the same calorie consumption split into 5 or 6 different meals throughout the day. It's said that you need a specific amount of proteins just to maintain your muscle mass. However, muscle mass can be also maintained through intermittent fasting, a process which doesn't focus specifically on protein intake. Remember, the growth hormone reaches unbelievable levels after 48 hours of fasting, so you can easily maintain your muscles without eating many proteins, or having protein bars or shakes.

As you already know, nothing is perfect and intermittent fasting is no exception. There are a few side effects that you need to worry about, like:

•hunger is perhaps the most common side effect of this way of eating, but the more you get used to IF, the less hunger you will feel

•beware of constipation, as when you eat less, you will not have to go to the toilet very often, so you can feel constipated at the beginning

•headaches should be expected when fasting. Food deprivation is a direct cause of these headaches. However, controlling your hunger and getting used to fasting, will be the best weapon to fight against these headaches

•during intermittent fasting, you might experience muscle cramps, heartburn, and dizziness

•in the case of athletic women, or those with very low body fat percentage, intermittent fasting may lead to a higher risk of irregular periods and lower chances of conception (so it reduces fertility for these women)

Chapter 6: Intermittent Fasting Types

There are so many different ways to practice Intermittent Fasting that this entire chapter is dedicated to just those methods. I will walk you through 10 specific and different methods for IF before ending with a section on how to make your choice. By the end of this chapter, if you've chosen to try IF, you should feel that your IF plans have direction and form, and you should be excited to implement these new plans into your daily routine.

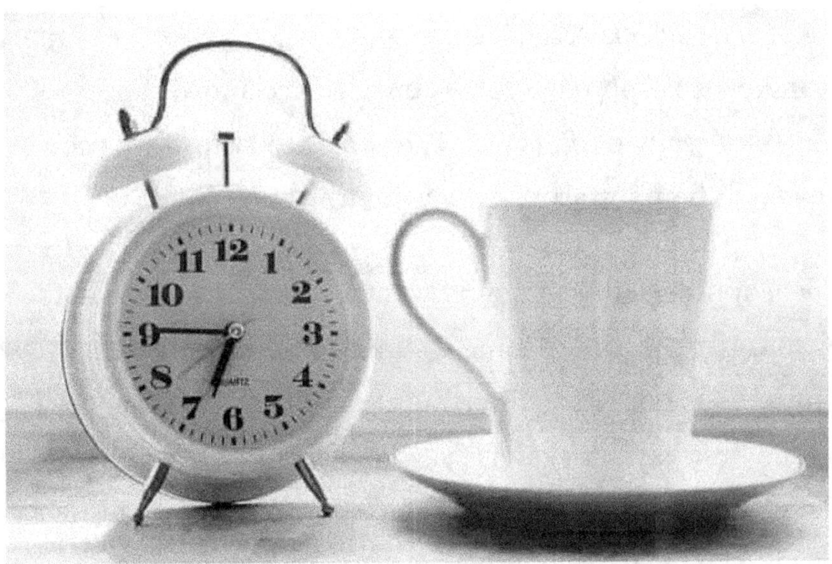

Explanation of Different Methods

Before you can start practicing Intermittent Fasting and incorporating it into your lifestyle, you'll have to know all the possibilities so you can choose the right one(s) for yourself, your goals, your habits, and your body/personality type. Read through the following 10 suggestions to find which methods sound most right to you.

Lean-Gains Method

The lean-gains method essentially focuses on the combined efforts of rigorous exercise, fasting, and a healthy diet. The fame surrounding this approach comes from its acclaimed success at turning fat directly into muscle. The goal is to fast within each day for 14-16 hours, starting when you wake up.

The ideal approach to lean-gains seems to be that you wake up and fast until 1 pm, doing some stretches and pre-workout warmups just before noon. Starting at noon, you would engage in training in whatever exercise you choose for an hour or less, ending with you breaking fast around 1 pm. Your meal at this time would be the largest of the day.

You would engage in your day as normal past then, as possible, eating again around 4 pm, then eating for the final time around 9 pm, giving yourself a ~15-hour fast until the next day at 1 pm. If you choose this approach yet feel a bit overwhelmed, you can work up to 15 hours, starting with a 13- or 14-hour fast only for the first week, building up to 15- or 16-hour fasting after that.

16:8 Method

16:8 method is one of the most popular methods among Intermittent Fasters. Essentially, you spend 16 hours within each day fasting, and the other 8 hours are your eating window. Most people try to choose their 8-hour eating window to be the times when they're primarily active. If you're a night person, feel free to make it a little later. Hold off eating during the daytime as much as possible then breakfast around 3 or 4 pm. For morning people, breakfast earlier, say, around 11 am, stopping food consumption by 7 pm.

16:8 is an incredibly flexible method that works for many different kinds of people. It's even flexible once you decide to try a particular fasting to eating window ratio. For example, if you don't seem to be jiving with the 11-7pm eating window, you can absolutely alter the next day to suit your needs better. Maybe try waiting until later in the day to breakfast! Try what you need to do, as long as you're keeping to that 16:8-hour ratio.

Whereas lean-gains method technically applies the same hourly ratio, it's much more strict regarding healthy diet and exercise regimen. 16:8 method does not need any type of exercise booster, but that's up to the practitioner. It is always best to try adding healthy dietary choices to one's IF eating schedule but don't try to restrict too many calories, as it can incorporate to feelings of lightheadedness and low energy. With 16:8, you can eat what you need and swap the hours around as desired.

14:10 Method

Similar to 16:8 method, 14:10 requires fasting and eating in varying degrees within each day. In this case, you would fast for 14 hours and engage in eating for a 10-hour window afterward. This method has the same flexibility as 16:8 in terms of what time of day it's arranged around, and how easy it is to troubleshoot. But it's additionally flexible in the sense that the eating window is two hours longer, accommodating people with more intense physical routines or daily demands, as well as people who simply need to eat a little later in the day to feel well.

20:4 Method

Whereas 14:10 method was an easier step down from 16:8 method, 20:4 method is definitely a step up in terms of difficulty. It's a more intense method certainly, for it requires 20 hours of fasting within each day with only a 4-hour eating window for the individual to gain all his or her nutrients and energy.

Most people who try this method end up having either one large meal with several snacks or they have two smaller meals with fewer snacks. 20:4 is flexible in that sense—the sense whereby the individual chooses how the eating window is divided amongst meals and snacks.

20:4 method is tricky, for many people instinctually over-eat during the eating window, but that's neither necessary nor is it healthy. People that choose 20:4 method should try to keep meal portions around the same size that they would normally have been without fasting. Experimenting on how many snacks are needed will be helpful as well with this method.

Many people end up working up to 20:4 from other methods, based on what their bodies can handle and what they're ready to attempt. Few start with 20:4, so if it's not working for you right away, please don't be too hard on yourself! Step it back to 16:8

and then see how soon you can get back to where you'd like to be.

The Warrior Method

The warrior method is quite similar to 20:4 method in that the individual fasts for 20 hours within each day and breaks fast for a 4-hour eating window. The difference is in the outlook and mindset of the practitioner, however. Essentially, the thought process behind warrior method is that, in ancient times, the hunter coming home from stalking prey or the warrior coming home from battle would really only get one meal each day. One meal would have to provide sustenance for the rest of the day, recuperative energy from the ordeal, and sustainable energy for the future.

Therefore, practitioners of warrior method are encouraged to have one large meal when they breakfast, and that meal should be jam-packed with fats, proteins, and carbs for the rest of the day (and for the days ahead). Just like with 20:4 method, however, it can sometimes be too intense for practitioners, and it's very easy to scale this one back in forcefulness by making up a method like 18:6 or 17:7. If it's not working, don't force it to work past two weeks, but do try to make it through a week to see if it's your stubbornness or if it's just a mismatch with the method.

12:12 Method

12:12 method is a little easier, along with the lines of 14:10, rather than 16:8 or 20:4. Beginners to Intermittent Fasting would do well to try this one right off the bat. Some people get 12 hours of sleep each night and can easily wake up from the fasting period, ready to engage with the eating window. Many people use this method in their lives without even knowing it.

To go about 12:12 method in your life, however, you'll want to be as purposeful about it as you can be. Make sure to be strict about your 12-hour cut-offs. Make sure it's working and feeling good in your body, and then you're invited to take things up a notch and try, say, 14:10 or maybe your own invention, like 15:11. As always, start with what works and then move up (or down) to what feels right (and even possibly better).

5:2 Method

5:2 method is popular among those who want to take things up a notch generally. Instead of fasting and eating within each day, these individuals take up a practice of fasting two whole days out of the week. The other 5 days are free to eat, exercise, or diet as desired, but those other two days (which can be consecutive or scattered throughout the week) must be strictly fasting days.

For those fasting days, it's not as if the individual can't eat anything altogether, however. In actuality, one is allowed to consume no more than 500 calories each day for this Intermittent Fasting method. I suppose these fasting days would be better referred to as "restricted-intake" days, for that is a more accurate description.

5:2 method is extremely rewarding, but it is also one of the more difficult ones to attempt. If you're having issues with this method, don't be afraid to experiment the next week with a method like 14:10 or 16:8, where you're fasting and eating within each day. If that works better for you, don't be ashamed to embrace it! However, if you're dedicated to having days "on" and days "off" with fasting and eating, there are other alternatives, too.

Eat-Stop-Eat (24-Hour) Method

The eat-stop-eat or 24-hour method is another option for people who want to have days "on" and "off" between fasting and eating. It's a little less intense than 5:2 method, and it's much more flexible for the individual, based on what he or she needs. For instance, if you need a literal 24-hour fast each week and that's it, you can do that. On the other hand, if you want a more flexible 5:2 method-type thing to happen, you can work with what you want and create a method surrounding those desires and goals.

The most successful approaches to the eat-stop-eat method have involved more strict dieting (or at the very least, cautious and healthy eating) during the 5 or 6 days when the individual engages in the week's free-eating window. For the individual to truly see success with weight loss, there will have to be some caloric restriction (or high nutrition focus) those 5 or 6 days, too, so that the body will have a version of consistency in health and nutrition content.

On the one or two days each week the individual decides to fast, there can still be highly-restricted caloric intake. As with 5:2 method, he or she can consume no more than 500 calories worth of food and drink during these fasting days so that the body can maintain energy flow and more.

If the individual engages in exercise, those workout days should absolutely be reserved for the 5 or 6 free-eating days. The same goes for 5:2 method. Try not to exercise (at least not excessively) on those days that are chosen for fasting. Your body will not appreciate the added stress when you're taking in so few calories. As always, you can choose to move up from eat-stop-eat to another method if this works easily and you're interested in something more. Furthermore, you can start with a strict 24-hour method and then move up to a more flexible eat-stop-eat approach! Do what feels right, and never be afraid to troubleshoot one method for the sake of choosing another.

Alternate-Day Method

The alternate-day method is similar to eat-stop-eat and 5:2 methods because it focuses on individual days "on" and "off" for fasting and eating. The difference for this method, in particular, is that it ends up being at least 2 days a week fasting, and sometimes, it can be as many as 4.

Some people follow very strict approaches to alternate-day method and literally fast every other day, only consuming 500 calories or less on those days designated for fasting. Some people, on the other hand, are much more flexible, and they tend to go for two days eating, one day fasting, two days eating, one day fasting, etc. The alternate-day method is even more flexible than eat-stop-eat in that sense, for it allows the individual to choose how he or she alternates between eating and fasting, based on what works for the body and mind the best.

The alternate-day method is like a step up from eat-stop-eat and 24-hour methods, especially if the individual truly alternates one-day fasting and the next day eating, etc. This more intense style of fasting works particularly well for people who are working on equally intense fitness regimens, surprisingly. People who are eating more calories a day than 2000 (which is true for a lot of bodybuilders and fitness buffs) will have more to gain from the alternate-day method, for you only have to cut back your eating on fasting days to about 25% of your standard caloric intake. Therefore, those fasting days can still provide solid nutritional support for fitness experts while helping them sculpt their bodies and maintain a new level of health.

Spontaneous Skipping Method

Alternate-day method and eat-stop-eat method are certainly flexible in their approaches to when the individual fasts and when he or she eats. However, none of those mentioned above plans are quite as flexible as spontaneous skipping method. Spontaneous skipping method literally only requires that the individual skip meals within each day, whenever desired (and when it's sensed that the body can handle it).

Many people with more sensitive digestive systems or who practice more intense fitness regimens will start their experiences with IF through spontaneous skipping method before moving on to something more intensive. People who have very haphazard daily schedules or people who are around food a lot but forget to eat will benefit from this method, for it works well with chaotic schedules and unplanned energies.

Despite that chaotic and unorganized potential, spontaneous skipping method can also be more structured and organized, depending on what you make of it! For instance, someone desiring more structure can choose which meal each day they'd like to skip. Let's say he chooses to skip breakfast each day. Then, his spontaneous skipping method will be structured around making sure to skip breakfast (a.k.a.—not to eat until at least 12 pm) daily. Whatever you need to do to make this method work, try it! This method is made for experimentation and adventurousness.

Crescendo Method

The final method worth mentioning is crescendo method, which is very well-suited for female practitioners (since their anatomies can be so detrimentally sensitive to high-intensity fasts). Essentially, this approach is made for internal awareness, gentle introductions, and gradual additions, depending on what works and what doesn't. It's a very active, trial-and-error type of method.

Through crescendo method, the individual starts by only fasting 2 or 3 days a week, and on those fast days, it wouldn't be a very intense fast at all. In fact, it wouldn't even be so strict that the individual would have to consume no more than 500 calories, like with 5:2, eat-stop-eat, and others. Instead, these "fasting" days would be trial periods for methods like 12:12, 14:10, 16:8, or 20:4. The remaining 4 or 5 days out of the week would be open eating-window periods, but again, the practitioner is encouraged to maintain a healthy diet throughout the week.

Crescendo method works extremely well for female practitioners because it enables them to see how methods like 14:10 or 12:12 will affect their bodies without tying them to the method hook, line, and sinker. It allows them to see what each method does to their hormone levels, their menstruation tendencies, and their mood swings. Therefore, the crescendo method encourages these people to be more in touch with their bodies before moving too quickly into something that could do serious anatomical and hormonal damage.

Crescendo method will work extremely well for overweight or diabetic practitioners, too, for it will allow them to have these same "trial period" moments with all the methods before choosing what feels and works best, based on each individual situation.

Making your Choice

When you make your choice from the 10 different options listed above, there are several things you'll want to keep in mind. First and foremost, amongst those things will be the fact that you can always choose another method (or a more flexible one to start with) in case something doesn't work as you'd hoped.

Ultimately, you'll also want to keep the following points in mind as you go about selecting your method: body type & abilities, lifestyle, daily tendencies, work routine, friends & family, and dietary choices. For all these considerations, remember what feels best to you, and remember to keep your goals with IF in mind at all times! If you ever feel like you're sacrificing your sanity or bodily health to attain these goals, go back to that step of troubleshooting, for you should never need to sacrifice those things to achieve any type of goals. Essentially, keep your eye on the prize and remember to choose what feels right and see what works from there.

Consider your body type and abilities. Think of how your body looks and feels and how much about it you'd like to change.

Think about how you react to food and what it looks like when you're hungry. Think about those things you view as your "limits" and how comfortable you are with pushing. Are you a fitness freak or a couch potato? Are you huskier or slimmer? Does your body hold onto fat or build muscle quickly? Do you retain water weight or not? Do you work out? Do you require a lot of water when you do? Consider all these things about your body and more, then compare them to the methods listed above. Compare them, too, to your overall goals with Intermittent Fasting to make sure that you're choosing a method that will help you actualize those goals as you conceive of them. If you're looking to lose weight quickly, try a method that works with days "on" and "off" between fasting and eating. If you're looking to build muscle, lean-gains method is probably the choice for you! If you're looking to boost your brain and heart, start with crescendo method and see where it takes you!

Consider your lifestyle. When do you normally wake up and how much sleep do you get on an average night? How hungry are you normally when you do wake up? How fast is your metabolism and when do you notice its peak? How do you make your living? Do you spend a lot of time in the car or on your feet or in an office? Are you constantly around other people or are you often alone? When you choose your method for Intermittent Fasting, make sure to consider all these lifestyle points. Maybe you wouldn't want to choose to time with a method that disallows you to eat when you normally need the most energy. Maybe you wouldn't want to choose a method that forces you to eat when you're supposed to be at work. Most of these methods have a degree of choice and flexibility, so when you do find one you like, remember that you don't have to put yourself in positions that go against your nature (or circadian rhythms) to achieve any of your goals. Stay flexible, keep your goals in mind, and respect the norms of your body!

Consider your daily tendencies. Do you eat mostly in the daylight hours or after the sun goes down? Do you go to work in the daytime or nighttime? Are you generally nocturnal, diurnal, or crepuscular? Do you have a lot of freedom and flexibility in your daily routines? Do you travel a lot for work? Do you spend a lot of time on the move? Do you have trouble remembering to eat? Are you the type of person that works out on the regular? Consider these themes in your life and more before you choose your method. Does it make sense for you to have low intake days where you consume 500 calories or less? Or does it make more sense for you to have extended periods in each day where you're just not eating based on your habits or tendencies or otherwise? Plan something that makes sense and respects your habits so that the transition into Intermittent Fasting is as easy and painless as possible.

Consider your work routine. Do you go to work in the morning or night? Are you allowed to eat at work? Do you work around food or in the food service industry? Do you work on your feet all day or by doing something strenuous? Do you receive purposeful or accidental exercise opportunities at work or are you just sitting in the same position all day? All these elements of your work routine will be important to consider as you decide which avenue of Intermittent Fasting to go down. You won't want to engage in a method like 20:4 if you're at work every day for incredibly short shifts. 20:4 works better for someone who works very long and distracting days. You won't want to try a method like 12:12 if part of your eating window involves being at work, when you're not allowed to eat at work. Remember to take your work life, routines, and restrictions into account when you go about making this choice, for you will make things much less harsh on yourself if you can look at this bigger picture from the beginning and planning stages.

Consider your friends, coworkers, and family. How loud are their opinions? Are their lives oriented toward health? Do they demean you a lot or make fun of your choices? Or are they encouraging all the time? Are these people your support system or are they your devils' advocates? Do you have the sense that they want to see you succeed? On the most basic level, are they nice to you and respectful of your choices? It might not seem that important, but the attitudes and supportive capacity of your friends, coworkers, and family can mean the world when you make a big choice like starting Intermittent Fasting in your life. Sometimes, people just don't want to see us succeed. They block our successes with jealousy, pride, ignorance, or arrogance. When friends and family act like this, it's better to choose a method that allows you to avoid discussing IF around them whatsoever. When friends and family are open and supportive, they shouldn't influence your choice that much at all; it's just when things are tenuous that you'll need to keep them (and your time around them) in consideration.

Finally, consider your dietary choices. Do you eat a lot of processed foods? Or do you eat a largely whole-foods, plant-based diet? Do you count calories? Do you cautiously skim nutrition facts? Are you looking for something specific like high fat, high fiber, or high protein? Are you hoping to change your diet entirely or are you trying to keep things the way they are? Are you willing to sacrifice items of your diet to actualize your goals? All these questions help determine which type of method you're going to be ready for. Essentially, if you're trying to change your diet entirely, a method with days "on" and days "off" will work best for you. In this case, try 5:2, alternate-day, eat-stop-eat, and spontaneous skip methods. However, if you don't want to change your diet that much at all, a method where you fast for periods within each day will be desirable instead.

Try methods like 20:4, 16:8, 14:10, or 12:12 for this type of situation.

As long as you make your selection with these 6 points in mind, you're sure to succeed with your Intermittent Fasting goals. You enable yourself to make the safest, smartest, best choice for your circumstances, and that's an incredible tool to use in so many different applications. In this case, it's a tool that will help keep you healthy, boost your brain, heal your heart, and shed that excess weight like melted butter!

As a reminder, your first choice still might not be the absolute right one, but by making the most educated choice possible, you're sure to start from a good place and learn a lot about yourself regardless. Make sure you have a runner-up method (or two!) that's easy to swap to just in case the first one doesn't seem to show progress. Work smarter, not harder! Plan ahead, do the research and know yourself. These are the truest steps to success that I know. And as always, don't be afraid to check with your doctor or nutritionist once the choice has been made. They'll be able to give you the final affirmation you need so you can get started on your new, healthy lifestyle with Intermittent Fasting in no time!

Chapter 7: What to Eat

We can distinguish 4 different categories for different types of drinks and effects they have on fasting:

- 0 kcal liquid foods that enhance the effects of fasting. Do not be afraid, during fasting periods when you will not have to touch food and therefore you will not consume meals, you will have the opportunity to drink non-caloric drinks, the important thing is that they are not sweetened. In this category we have foods such as vinegar, coffee, green tea, black tea, multivitamin supplements (which I recommend taking with vegetables and not on an empty stomach), *WATER*. Stimulants, such as caffeine, which mediates the production of norepinephrine which mobilizes glucose stores and increasing the *ADP / ATP* ratio in turn activates *AMPK / PPAR* which is enough to let us know that they are all events that enhance the mobilization of acids fats and catabolic processes involved in fasting. As for water, which is often not considered too much, drinking a good quantity of water at one time causes a rise in pressure mediated by the norepinephrine, which reconnected to what has been said about stimulants makes us guess that it has a very important.

- Caloric liquid foods that potentiate the effects of fasting. Among the foods that we can consider non-zero calories, we certainly find famous BCAAs (even if they are powdered, they must be dissolved in water and therefore we consider them liquid), branched amino acids, even if they supply calories to our body, for a direct effect on the limitation of muscle catabolism (they are gluconeogenesis, they are used in place of the amino acids obtained from the destruction of muscle to produce glucose) they bring benefits for fasting. Another "surprise" food in this category is coconut oil, although it is a fat and therefore very caloric, it does not interrupt carbohydrate fasting, it activates the metabolic pathways that promote lipid oxidation, but being mainly composed of acids Medium chain fats (MCTs) will be very quickly, and likely directed to the mitochondria rather than being accumulated as fat. Other similar foods are ghee or clarified butter, largely composed of MCT fat.

- o kcal liquid foods that block the effects of fasting (or have no effect on it). There is not much to say about this category of liquids, because it should not even exist since there are practically no calorie foods that block the fast, but only foods that have no effect on it, although not interrupting it, we could think of sweeteners, but from several researches recently published, it has been noted that they have an (indirect) influence on the release of insulin, mediated by the perception of "sweet taste". Obviously a few drops in coffee or tea will not block the fast, but it will not have positive effects either, they are "neutral". An example of drinks are "zero" sodas, which if you follow Martin Berkhan, you know you can take in quantity.

- Caloric liquid foods that block the effects of fasting. Practically the most intuitive category; sugary drinks and liquid foods that bring more than 50 kcal per 100g, if you like a drop of milk in coffee, it will not be the one to block it (provided it is a drop and not milk coffee). For solid foods we have a greater limitation, practically there are foods that block fasting (calories) and foods that enhance their effects (calorie or limited calorie <50 kcal per 100g).

- Fasting foods (calories). All known and intuitive foods, cereals, sweets, dairy products, oils etc. etc., in short, all categories of foods that are excluded from fasting (using a little common sense you can easily guess). Foods that enhance its effects (calorie or limited calories <50 kcal per 100g): It is an interesting category, since we find very interesting foods, such as meat, for those who practice a PSMF (Protein Spared Modified Fast) it is practically a fast in which they only take proteins to limit muscle catabolism and spices; Among these we have cinnamon, black pepper, chili pepper, turmeric. They are all spices that act on the catabolism factors (for example, the chili pepper slightly increases the metabolism, making sure that the calories ingested are less than those needed to digest it, on an empty stomach it is a BOMB to enhance its effects).

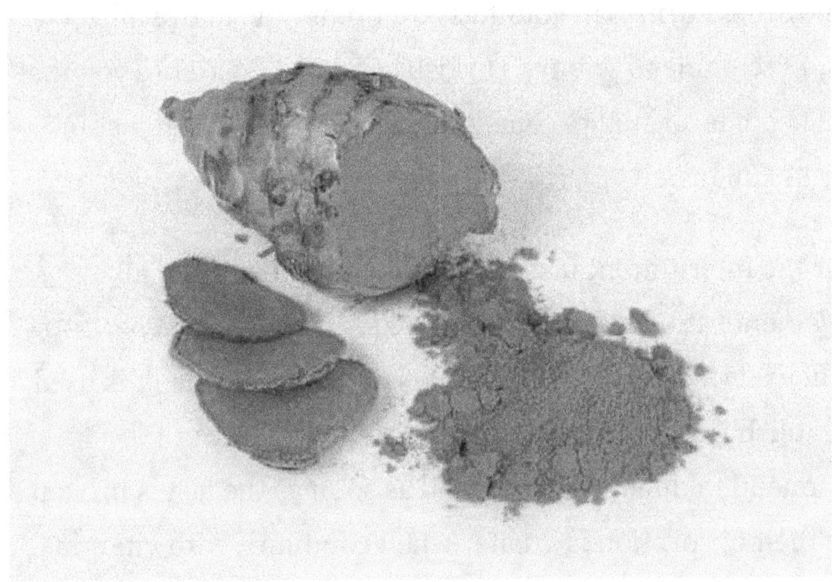

Now that you know how fasting is "created", you can well try experimenting with combinations of the various foods that will make it much more effective (and pleasant, like fasting coffee for example). An example is that of the famous "Bulletproof coffee", MCT fats such as coconut oil or ghee (clarified butter) dissolved in hot coffee (or blended together), it may seem crap but I assure you it is a unique goodness, the foam that forms is a pleasure. But also combinations like mint and cinnamon coffee, or mint and vanilla tea, are all tastes that we Westerners are not used to and can seem strong or disgusting; instead in the Far East it has been used for centuries, if in fact you are looking for some 0 kcal recipe with coffee or tea, you will be amazed at how simple it is to enjoy these drinks in countless different (and above all good) ways, I recommend you try Turkish coffee, and I assure you that it will become a ritual to remain on an empty stomach just to savor its full taste!

As for the intermittent fasting supplement, practically all supplements at 0 kcal or that involve less than 50 kcal per 100g are allowed (it is an office value, it is not a magic rule, it is used to establish a range). Multivitamins are also fine, but I recommend taking them with food as soon as the fast is broken since their absorption is greater when combined with vitamins with high biological availability (such as those found in vegetables). More of this goes to isotonic drinks, there is no problem as long as the *TOTAL* calories of the drink that are under the fateful 50 kcal, be sure to check the value of kcal you take per serving.

Chapter 8: Commons Mistakes and How to Fix them

Busting the Myths

- **Intermittent fasting will decrease metabolic rate.** Fasting is proven to increase your metabolic rate when done the right way. You will benefit from a leaner weight loss that helps retain the most muscle mass possible.

- **It is not OK to skip breakfast.** Contrary to popular belief, breakfast is not sacred or more important than any other meal. It is neutral. You can take it or leave it. Skipping breakfast won't add weight since you take in zero calories. Eating breakfast won't rev up the metabolic rate any more than another meal. So, go ahead and let go of the myth that you can't skip breakfast if this is what is holding you back.

- **You need to eat small meals throughout the day.** There is no basis to the belief that snacking boosts metabolism. Current research shows that snacking can contribute to fatty liver disease. It's perfectly fine and healthy to eat reasonably sized nutritious meals. Although widely accepted as a

method of weight loss, there is no basis for the idea
that eating multiple small meals throughout the day
is a good strategy. It may serve the process of
decreasing overall calorie consumption, but it's not a
fast-track to weight loss. This eating pattern
introduces a constant supply of calories and does not
give the body time to recover and regenerate.

Common Intermittent Fasting Mistakes to Avoid

Tea and coffee don't count, but cream and sugar do!
Don't make the mistake of thinking added fats and sugars don't
matter. If you choose to undertake intermittent fasting, follow
the rules. Don't think that you can sneak some cream into your
coffee or some sugar into your tea. If you want to do this, and
you are ready to take a break from your fast for whatever reason,
then treat yourself. Just don't call it a fasted period, because it
isn't if your body is putting out the effort to process the fat or
sugar consumed. Even small amounts will throw your system off
and the metabolic process of your body will be altered. Any
amount, no matter how small, of protein or carbohydrate will
trigger your metabolism and begin the myriad processes put
into effect once digestion is activated. Once these processes

begin, you are not fasting. Get used to drinking your tea plain and your coffee black while fasting.

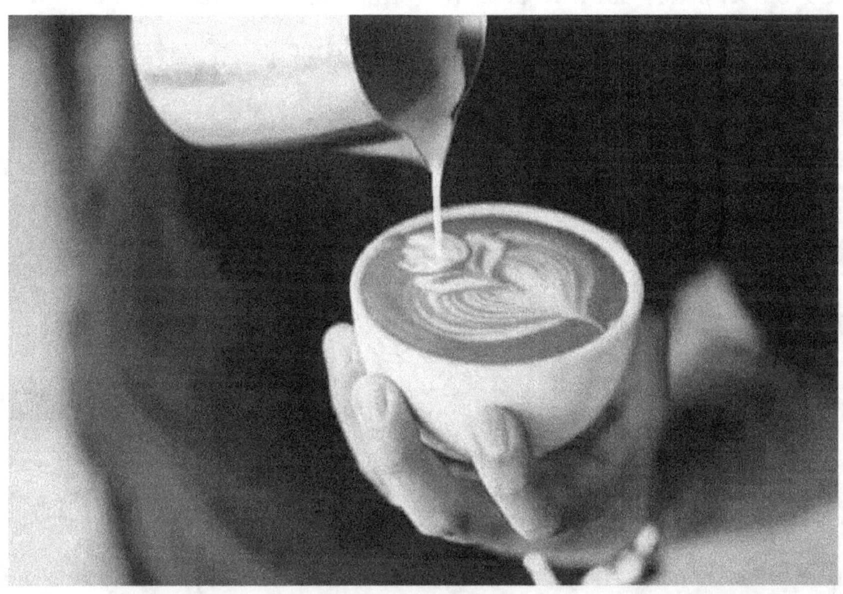

Don't drink too much coffee. You guessed it, this was coming. Of course, whatever amount of coffee you decide is right for you must be black. Some women seem to fuel their lives on coffee. This may be fine, but be careful while you are fasting to observe if the way your body responds is different. Drinking Black coffee while fasting is somewhat controversial. Some people love it for its fat-burning effect, while others say that caffeine will set off your insulin response. Unfortunately, it has the impact of effectively taking you out of fasting mode. It's perfectly safe to drink black coffee during the fasting window, but be careful about how much. Make sure to compensate with extra water, because coffee deprives your system of fluids.

Coffee is considered a diuretic, which is a compound that causes your body to produce a ton of urine. Is it because caffeine increases blood flow through the kidneys? No one has honestly taken the time to find out and published studies. If you are not careful, your body can suffer from dehydration. It's less of a risk to drink coffee while you are eating because you actually receive large amounts of water from foods.

Caffeine is another question. Research indicates it can contribute to burning fat and suppress the appetite. That's all fine and good but don't consume so much that you get a buzz from it, as this may mean it triggers the insulin response you want to avoid while in the fasted state. Be careful with decaf as well. It still has diuretic properties and contains significantly more caffeine than black tea or green tea. The bottom line with coffee, regular or decaf, is that you do not want to become dehydrated.

Drink enough water. Do not make the mistake of not drinking enough water! No matter how much coffee or tea you are drinking while fasting, you need to be sure to drink plenty of water. You'll hear a ton of different advice on the exact amount needed every day, but base it on your activity level. Keep in mind this is a minimum amount. Few studies indicate that you can drink too much water, so don't be afraid to drink more than you normally would.

Remember that your body is not getting any water from food during the **fasted** state. It makes it more crucial you don't deprive your system of needed water. This is probably the single most fundamental part of intermittent fasting. It will not work without water. You cannot fast without drinking water. You can certainly also drink tea, and whatever amount of coffee you can handle, but don't forget to drink water. This is true of the time you spend in the **fed** state as well, but it's twice as important not to become dehydrated while fasting. All the cellular regeneration and rebuilding that is going on requires water. The waste products in your system that need to be released throughout the process of fasting require being flushed out, which calls for water.

If you make the mistake of not drinking water, you risk the possibility of becoming sick or having adverse symptoms including, but not limited to, headaches, nausea, lightheadedness or muscle pain. In summary, make sure to drink lots of water during your fasting window. It will serve the purpose of keeping you well-hydrated and help you detoxify at the same time. You can incorporate other no-calorie drinks as well, including herbal tea, apple cider vinegar, or mineral supplements. Start small and make sure any additives have zero calories and they don't upset your stomach. Be especially careful with mineral or vitamin supplements, as they can cause nausea while fasting.

Don't make the mistake of using intermittent fasting as an excuse to eat only unhealthy food. Intermittent fasting offers many great health benefits and it would be a significant mistake to counter-act the benefits by choosing to eat only processed food. Intermittent fasting can help mitigate the effects of a bad diet, but it's not a reason to give yourself a free pass to go and eat all the junk you can lay your hands on.

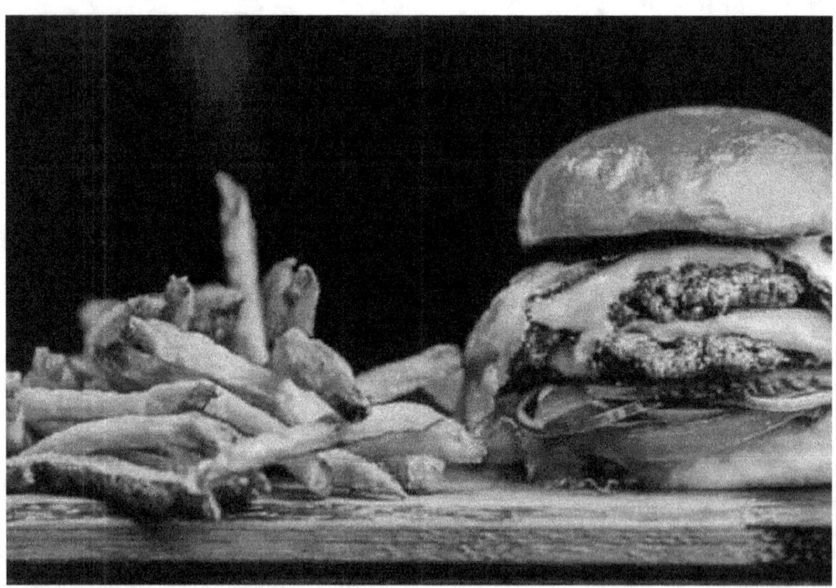

Intermittent fasting does help increase your metabolic flexibility and your ability to handle the occasional turkey dinner. It can even assist with occasional all you can eat buffet. Don't think it gives you a free pass to eat only junk food all the time. That's a sure recipe for disaster and not at all how intermittent fasting is intended to be used. It leads to even more bad eating habits, which is what you are trying to correct.

While intermittent fasting is a physical process, allowing our bodies the opportunity to repair and rejuvenate, it's also a mental exercise. It's a choice to fast we are making out of our own free will. When you try to be too militant or rigidly follow the clock, you're taking the choice away and inviting burnout. And, you're also bringing the possibility of failure to the table. If you normally don't eat until after 8 pm but you don't finish eating until 8:15, don't sweat the small stuff. The extra 15-minutes won't undo your efforts.

Fasting is also not the same as depriving ourselves of food. If you're hungry, famished and out of sorts, then eat! That may be what you need today and tomorrow you can try again to see if the process will go more smoothly. It's important that it fits into your life in a way that works for you. It's not worth forcing. Force makes it something to dread. It's not an area of life you want to tie yourself to a rigid and unforgiving regimen.

As you practice intermittent fasting more, to the point it becomes a part of your life, you'll start to learn the difference between the _ghrelin hormonal cycles of hunger_ that pass easily and the very real need to eat. Don't push yourself too fast. Find a way to do it that works for you where you can forgive yourself, celebrate your successes and forgive your mistakes. The point is to become healthier and happier, not guilty because you've let yourself down.

Guilt never does anyone any good.

Don't try to be so strict about intermittent fasting that you take the fun and experimental joy out of the process. You'll be missing out on the best part. The key to success is to find the right fit for you, not to fit yourself to a rigid program.

Don't make the mistake of not eating enough during the eating window.

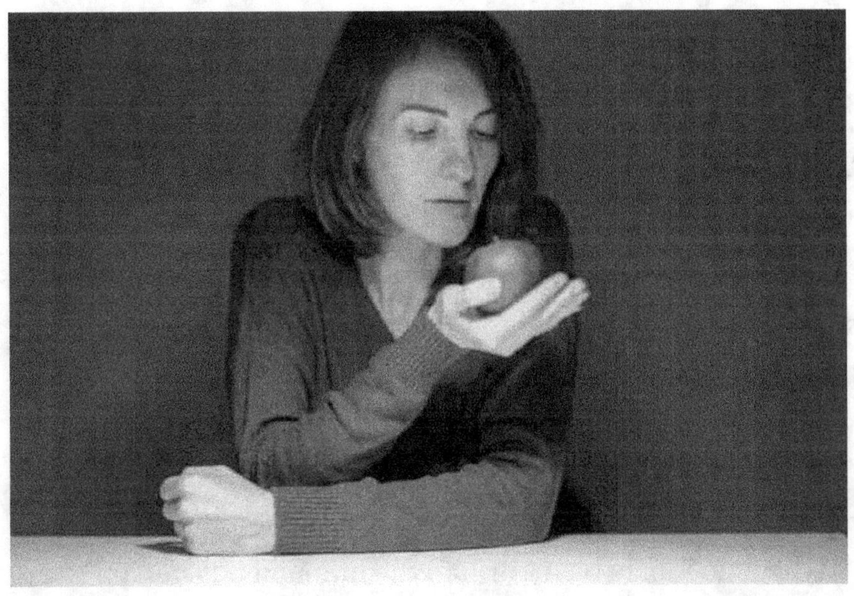

While intermittent fasting is effective and useful when practiced in conjunction with a weight loss goal, it's not, in and of itself, a diet. It's a mistake to use intermittent fasting as a form of purposeful, targeted calorie restriction. Intermittent fasting gives your body time to repair and clean out the cellular junk that's hanging around.

It leads to better function of all your body's systems, and it's important to support this with enough food to replenish and rebuild. Choose good, healthy, whole foods with lots of nutrient density and your body will get better at signaling when you have had enough. You will get better at listening to your body.

Transition slowly. Once people are introduced to intermittent fasting and find out about how great it is with its many benefits, they are eager to dive in. Instead of easing in and slowly transitioning in a way that is right for their bodies, they dive straight in, trying for long 6 to 18-hour fasts. Don't make this mistake! It can lead to overwhelming hunger, frustration and a quick end to the trial of intermittent fasting.

Intermittent fasting is a powerful tool to help your body rest and repair that's been used throughout many cultures in human history. While it may be natural to the human body, it won't be natural to your body if you haven't spent a lifetime practicing the method. It can be a lifelong practice, but only if you give yourself time to adjust.

Chapter 9: Intermittent Fasting Tips

At this point, you likely know which intermittent fasting strategy you're going to employ or which ones you're going to try deciding between since there truly *are* so many options, so it's time to start thinking of how to put your plan into action. While intermittent fasting can seem, to some, much less daunting than an entire diet change, it is just as intense as becoming vegan from being a meat-eater for others. That being said, no matter which camp you fall into, you'll likely need a few pointers for the adjustment period.

The gist of this chapter is to give you the information you need to make the transition into your first (or next) intermittent fast as easy and painless as it can be. You'll be provided with tips to help establish a new routine as well as informational tidbits of what to expect, what to do and what not to do, what to look out for and, for worst-case scenario moments, when to quit.

Before the chapter is finished, you will also be guided through common mistakes in the transition to intermittent fast. The hope is that you'll then be able to avoid such instances in your own experience as you decide how and when to move forward with IF yourself. You'll also be exposed to ways to "protect" against potential hiccups in the plan. Simply put, the more forethought, the better; the more you're mentally and emotionally ready for, the more successful your adventure with intermittent fasting will be overall. Let's make our way into getting started!

Transitional Tips

When you're about to begin your process of intermittent fasting, you'll need to have a few tricks up your sleeve to make the transition as painless as possible, and that's what this section is all about. First of all, make sure you do have some sort of method planned. Pick that plan and stick with it, at least for the first week. Next, do any extra research you may need to do, considering your body type and any diseases or disorders that you may have. This extra bit of research may be game-changing for you, in terms of making sure your transition into IF has no disruptions or toxic effects for your body type. If it's necessary at this point, check with your doctor to ensure that you're on the right track and that the method you've chosen poses no harm to you.

Something else you can do before start IF, is to look at your diet ahead of time and adjust things to be a little easier. As I mentioned before, a diet composed of primarily processed foods may pose complications for the individual during the detoxification period. As you can, start to replace processed foods, with whole foods (fruits, vegetables, grains, nuts, seeds, etc.) that support your health and healing. Additionally, as you plan which method you'll undertake, you can go into more detail and make sure your feasting is packed with the right nutrients between fast periods. Calculate the calories you'll need for each fast, the macronutrients you'll need to refuel, and the training you anticipate you'll be able to handle. The more forethought, the better.

When it comes to that first day of getting started in the intermittent fast lifestyle, the following pieces of advice will help to make things flow with ease. First of all, on the evening before, don't eat a late dinner, and don't eat after dinner. Make sure to have lots of drinks on hand for the fasting process ahead. Healthy and Imagine that night before that you're beginning your fast at sundown or after that early dinner. Then, when you go to sleep and wake up in the morning, you've already done almost 12 hours of fasting. At that point, delay your breakfast the next morning, and you can easily achieve 12 hours if not 14 of fasting right off the bat.

During this waiting period, have as many IF-safe drinks as needed, and then, when the eating window comes (if you choose a method that involves an eating window or at least if you try this day-1 transition guide), engage in eating, but don't snack too much. The following days, whether they involve eating windows or not, try to cut out snacks more often to help your body adjust. Other things you can do before and during your transition to IF include skipping breakfasts habitually or simply delaying them, having earlier dinners, or substituting snacks for smoothies.

Help for Routine-Setting

After the first few days, you may need a little help getting the routine affirmed and established, and the following pieces of advice are attuned to help with that exact problem. To assist in routine-setting, remember to keep things slow and simple, especially at the beginning of your process. Don't push yourself too hard and keep your expectations for the fast (and on yourself) realistic and grounded.

It could be that you've tried to start with a method that's too disruptive of your standard routine. It's much more productive to transition into something that's a somewhat "logical" extension of your daily activities.

What to Expect

When you begin intermittent fasting, there are several things you should expect from your experience, regardless of whether they're helpful or not. The points below will walk you through those details to prepare you for what's to come.

First of all, mornings may be completely different for you. You will likely find that your mornings become filled with energy or completely lethargic, depending on whether you were a morning or night person beforehand. Furthermore, you may experience your worst hunger pangs during the morning time, but this element is also affected by whether you're a morning or night person. Finally, coffee will become your best friend, if it's not already. Mornings may be the most serious times of fasting for you, and even if they're not fasting periods, you're still going to need that infamous morning juice (coffee, or at least something caffeinated that similarly kick-starts metabolism) to get you through the day as it is now, with less food in it.

Certain things will increase. During your initial transition period into intermittent fasting, your abilities to plan and organize are liable to massively and noticeably increase. You might find that scheduling your fast into your week feels impossible before you begin, but after the first few days, it will become more second-nature to organize and think in this way. Additionally, you will almost certainly become more mindful of the world around you, of your internal feelings, and of how food truly affects you. As one final note, recall all the potential benefits of intermittent fasting. Remind yourself of what you're working to grow in yourself, and you're sure to be propelled through the hard times.

Other things will decrease. The most common goal of intermittent fasting is to lose weight (yay!), and that will almost assuredly happen for every IF practitioner. That weight is bound to decrease with the appropriate application of intermittent fasting and healthy diet, given your body type and physical needs. Furthermore, you may lose sleep, at least during the first two weeks' detoxification period, which is detailed more in the next paragraph. Although sleep may be difficult, it will settle back into a normal pattern, and if you always have troubles with sleep, you might even find that you have the easiest, most restful sleep of your life while you're intermittently fasting.

During a period of the first two or so weeks, you will definitely go through a detoxification period. You will get stinky, moody, cranky, and tired. You will feel weird bursts of energy and then nothing at all. If you're working out as you practice intermittent fasting, you might find that your workouts during the first two weeks are especially exhausting or unproductive. You might have an emotional moment or two, but after these first two weeks, those powerful side-effects should go away, for they're all a part of the detox associated with the transition. You have to get through the rough patch to reap the rewards, however, so stick with the process and fight through those crunchy, harsh times.

You'll be thankful you pushed through, no matter how smelly you may get.

You may also experience somewhat negative side-effects, which will be detailed further in the section titled "What to Lookout For," which appears later in this chapter.

Finally, your relationship with food will become entirely different. It may take a couple of days — it may even take the entire detox period to get it right to settle into eating the *right amount* during your eating windows. At first, you might have trouble with either eating too much or not enough when it's time to eat, but you will be urged to work through any food dependency issues by this process regardless of how often and how much you eat. During times of fast, one can't help but consider with new eyes how food, hunger, and hangry feelings affect one's relationship with others and the world.

What to Do/What not to Do

When it comes down to it, knowing concisely what to do and what not to do will be the informational backbone to your success with intermittent fasting.

What to do includes:

- Start slow

- Track your progress

- Live normally, otherwise
  - Especially in times of fast, work and play are especially distracting when you're hungry!

- Help to suppress hunger with drinks like mineral water and with gum

- Keep tabs on your hormonal health
  - As a woman, it is especially important that you perform this work to troubleshoot IF in your life.

- Focus on fats when you eat (*without* making fat consumption your main goal)

On the other hand, **what not to do** includes:

- Don't start too hard and fast
  - Ease into it!

- Don't give up after just a week
  - This is a big no-no unless you display warning signs and worst-case-scenario markers.

- Don't diet too fiercely

- Don't work out too much

- Don't continue to intermittently fast even after you display warning signs

- Don't constantly eat during the eating windows
  - Don't forget that your body still needs breaks in eating to digest!

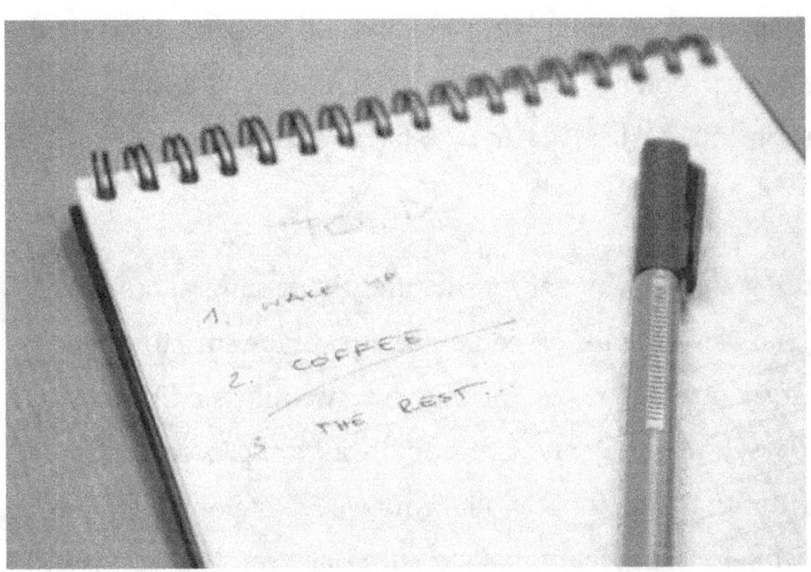

What to Lookout for

As you engage with intermittent fasting, there may be warning signs that your body is not benefitting from the process at hand. You'll have to be very keen and conscious of these warning signs, for if they appear, alterations will need to be made if your success and health are the goals (as they should be!). Overall, look out for warning signs like constant headaches, tiredness without the ability to sleep, dizziness, lightheadedness, or constant sleeping. While some of these elements can be signals that adjustments in the process are all that's needed, if you had any of these problems before trying IF and they've gotten *worse* as you continued with IF, you may have reached a quitting point.

Something else to look out for includes those general hunger pangs, but as we've discussed before, just make sure to ride those urges out like waves, for they surely will pass. Check in with yourself mentally and emotionally as you proceed with intermittent fasting, too, for your knowledge of yourself will be the most helpful aspect of making sure that your process is healthy for you. The process of intermittent fasting is one that can be easily abused and twisted into something that's unhealthy, but the better you know yourself, and the more you seek growth in this effort, the better off you'll be when it comes to IF.

When to Quit

Since you're female, you are a bit more likely to experience worst-case-scenario intermittent fasting moments than a male would be, but when you do come up against these scenarios, do not doubt that it is truly time for you to stop. Pushing beyond this point means your life stands at risk, and no fitness regime is worth that price. Do not take these worst-case-scenario warnings lightly.

Worst-case-scenario warnings include:

- Burning in the pit of your stomach
  - This sensation is a likely sign of gastritis or something even worse.

- Vomiting even when you've hardly eaten
  - You could have gastric irritation, an imbalance of electrolytes, or something more dangerous.

- Fainting
  - This issue is especially worrisome if it becomes habitual.

- Feeling a pain in your stomach or chest

- Experiencing diarrhea

- o   Diarrhea is troubling because can contribute to dehydration and imbalance of electrolytes if not noticed and fixed in time.

- Worrying period symptoms
  - o   such as: complete loss of period, excessive bleeding, or spotting when you're not supposed to be

Chapter 10: Why Intermittent Fasting Is Ideal for Women Over 50

There are many benefits to intermittent fasting that make it ideal for women as they age. Not only do women struggle to lose weight as they get older, and their metabolism slows down, but they also are more prone to many age-related and weight-related diseases. In this chapter, we will go point-by-point on some of the best reasons to choose this lifestyle.

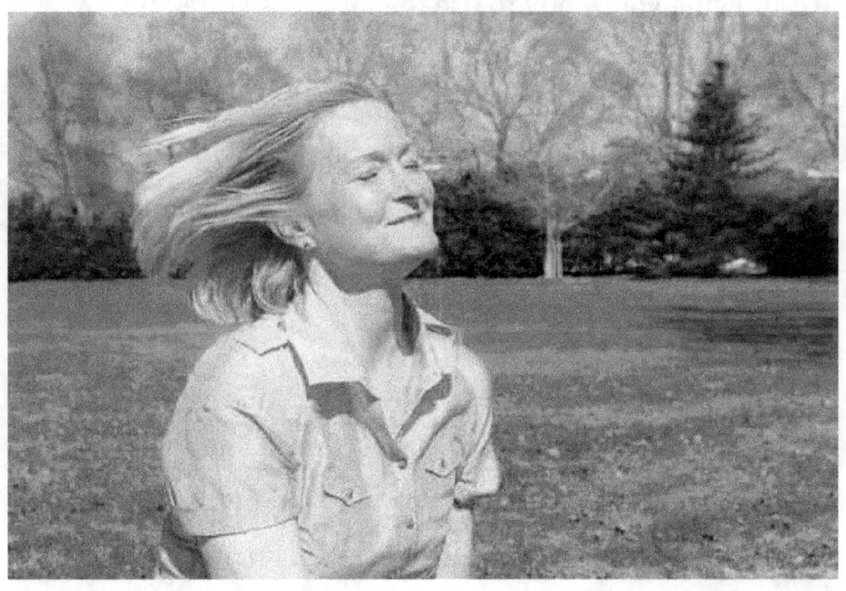

Weight Loss

While many people try diet after diet to lose weight, only to be disappointed, you can expect to find much more success with intermittent fasting. After all, while the human body is usually forced to be burning off the food regularly we have eaten, when you are in a fasted state, you can instead work on burning off your body fat. In the past, it was natural to go long periods without eating while working for the day. In today's modern society, we take a break for lunch and often for a snack as well, which only impedes weight loss. But, with fasting, you can eat the same number of calories and still lose weight, all because you are allowing your body to use the fat it has stored up.

Multiple studies conducted on intermittent fasting have found it much more effective than a variety of popular dieting and weight loss options, even when a person doesn't reduce their caloric intake.

Metabolic Reset

Many women, as they age, experience reduced metabolism. This is partly due to the natural aging process, and partly due to damaging the metabolism over the decades. Frequent crash dieting, poor sleep, overworking, poor health, and more can all damage your metabolism, thus preventing you from losing weight. But, by merely practicing intermittent fasting, you can reset and boost your metabolism, not only allowing you to lose weight but also helping you to feel healthier and maintain healthy lean muscle as you age.

Increase Human Growth Hormone

Hormones play an essential role in human health, something of which women are exceptionally aware of as they age. But many women are unaware of how to take advantage of the human growth hormone, also known as HGH. As this name implies, this hormone affects growth, but that is not all! This hormone is vital for bone health and density, cellular growth and regeneration, tissue health, and muscle mass. As women age, they tend to lose muscle mass, bones become thin and brittle, and cells begin to decay, increasing the speed of aging: all things that an increased level of HGH hormone can help improve.

When your body is in a fasted state, it leads to a boost in a natural increase in the HGH hormone. Studies have proven that this hormone can rise to five times its average level during a fast, meaning you can experience great full-body benefits to your health.

While it can be harmful if you experience a rise of this nature in many of your hormones, the same is not true of the human growth hormones. Studies have found that it is perfectly safe, even when it rises to this degree and higher. This is especially true since people naturally experience their HGH levels lowering as they age.

Convert your Body Fat

Many people are unaware, but there are two types of body fat, white and brown. This fat is not created equal. Just as there is healthy and unhealthy cholesterol, there is also sturdy and unhealthy body fat. The white fat, which is what builds up as people gain excess weight, is damaging to health, contributes to aging, and leads to disease.

On the other hand, brown body fat is vital in protecting the body's inner organs and maintaining health. When you practice intermittent fasting, it not only helps you lose weight, but it can also actively convert your unhealthy white fat to healthy brown fat. As if that weren't good enough, brown fat also helps burn off white fat, meaning that the more brown fat you have, the more you will burn off excess white body fat.

Improve Muscle Health

Many people get excited about the temporary weight reduction they experience when trying the crash diet. That is until they stop losing weight and eventually give up on a diet. But, most of the weight loss people achieve on these diets is not fat loss but water weight and muscle weight. Muscle weighs more than fat, so even a small amount of muscle loss can make a big difference on the scale.

As crash diets promote malnutrition, it naturally leads to muscle loss, which negatively affects your health and strength as you age. After all, your muscles are in much more than your arms. They are surrounding your entire body, and even your heart is a muscle! As you lose muscle, your health and energy will be dramatically affected, and it is essential to regain this as you age if you want to improve your health. Thankfully, studies have found that when compared to dieting, intermittent fasting not only leads to more weight loss than dieting, but it also causes much less muscle loss. This means your muscles will become much healthier, especially if you actively workout while you practice fasting.

Boosted Energy

The mitochondria, which are within our mitochondrial cells, are the powerhouse of the cell. It is the mitochondria that allow us to use a variety of fuel sources from the food we eat as fuel, as well as ketones. While other cells in the body may only be able to utilize one or two fuel types for energy, the mitochondrial is incredibly versatile to be able to use all kinds of fuel. When you fast for longer periods (or are on a low-carb/ketogenic diet), your body begins to produce ketones, which are then used to cross the blood-brain barrier and fuel the brain in the absence of glucose. But that is not all. When you are in this fasted state of ketosis, the body will also increase the number of mitochondrial cells within your body, replacing non-mitochondrial cells with mitochondrial cells, allowing for more of your cells to be fueled by any fuel source.

Since the mitochondrial fuel ninety percent of the human body, by increasing the number of these cells, you can naturally increase your energy. Not only will your physical energy increase, but your mental functioning and energy will, as well. This is great news for many people who lose energy as they age.

Reduce Insulin Resistance

Insulin is perhaps the most well-known hormone, as the number of people diagnosed with diabetes only continues to rise. But insulin does not only affect people with diabetes but for everyone. This hormone, produced by the pancreas, is released after eating to allow the cells to absorb and utilize glucose as an energy source. But, often, our sensitivity to insulin decreases as we age or put on weight. The cells can become resistant to insulin, which leads to them being unable to absorb the glucose we have ingested. Over time, this causes a buildup of glucose in the bloodstream and, ultimately, diabetes if it is left untreated.

However, whether you have insulin resistance or already have been diagnosed with type II diabetes, you don't have to allow your condition to worsen. You can treat your insulin resistance directly at the source, and in the process, improve the absorption of glucose by your cells. Many people can lower the severity of their insulin resistance or diabetes, and some are even able to treat it completely.

Multiple controlled studies have found that intermittent fasting can both treat insulin resistance and lower blood glucose levels. Some studies have found that intermittent fasting can even be as effective, if not more effective, than dieting for lowering blood glucose levels.

Reduce Excess and Chronic Inflammation

Inflammation plays an essential role in human health. Without inflammation, we would be the victim of any germ or bacteria that attempted to leave our body. This is why people with a compromised immune system can get sick and pass away so easily.

But, while it might be important to have a functioning immune system that will increase inflammation when we are sick or injured, sometimes we develop excess or chronic inflammation, which is also detrimental to our health. Sadly, cases of excessive and chronic inflammation are becoming more wide-spread due to environmental pollutants, overwork, poor diet, sleep deficiencies, and more. When this happens, the chronic inflammation no longer protects a person from diseases but instead predisposes them to more infection. For instance, studies have found that increased levels of inflammation can lead to heart disease, cancer, rheumatoid arthritis, and much more.

However, you don't have to accept the occurrence of excessive and chronic inflammation helplessly. Studies on the matter have found that intermittent fasting can drastically reduce chronic inflammation levels. One study found that within as little time as a month, participants' inflammation levels were drastically reduced. Another study specifically found that you can achieve these results simply by completing a daily twelve-hour fast for thirty days.

Increase Neural Cells

It is important to take care of brain health as we age, especially as the levels of Alzheimer's disease, Parkinson's disease, and other neurodegenerative diseases are on the rise. But, one way that intermittent fasting can help guard against and treat all brain-related diseases is by increasing the production and repair of neural cells. This is important, as these diseases all cause these vital brain cells to become damaged or stunted overtime.

The result is that if you begin practicing intermittent fasting regularly now, you can reduce your risk of developing a neurological disease in the future. Or, if you already have one, you may be able to reduce symptoms or halt its progression. This is amazing news, as neurological diseases are incredibly hard to treat, even with modern medicine. Studies have specifically shown intermittent fasting to increase cell growth and repair in the cortex, hippocampus, basal forebrain, and nervous system. Along with the decreased risk of disease and disease progression, you can also expect to experience increased mental energy, better focus, improved memory, and a stabilized mood.

Boost Cellular Health

As we age, our cells themselves also age and decrease in age, which is the aging process that we are all so familiar with. But there is a process known as autophagy that can reduce the aging of the cell, and therefore help slightly reduce aging and significantly increase health. There is no method to stop or reverse aging itself, but you can stop and reverse the aging of the cells. The autophagy process causes old, damaged, and dying cells to be replaced with younger and healthier cells, allowing you to maintain health. The process of autophagy is critical for maintaining homeostasis, and if it is malfunctioning, it leads to increased aging and disease.

Researchers have long studied this process, even going to far as to search for drugs that can induce the process of autophagy to treat people with chronic and terminal illnesses. But you can induce autophagy without drug treatments with intermittent fasting. Studies have found that by activating the autophagy process, intermittent fasting can even help your vital stem cells to regenerate themselves.

Lessen Oxidative Stress

Toxins cause oxidative stress. We can develop these toxins when we breathe in poor quality air, don't sleep well, eat poor quality food, apply damaging substances to our skin, and much more. We even develop this oxidative stress when our cells convert fuel to energy, meaning that even if we live in a clean environment, sleep perfectly, and only eat organic food, we would still develop oxidative stress, thereby causing damage to our cells. As our cells develop this damage from oxidative stress, we slowly lose our health and energy, producing an increased risk of disease.

However, studies have shown that intermittent fasting not only increases the rate our cells develop oxidative stress, but it also increases our body's natural antioxidants to fight against this damage directly.

Improve Mental Well-Being

Poor mental health is becoming more common than ever, with over forty-million Americans suffering from one form of mental illness or another, and many others struggling with short-term depression and anxiety. One of the most common causes of disability in middle-aged Americans (as well as those who are young) is chronic severe depression. Yet, a majority of these people never seek professional help.

While I urge you always to seek professional help for your mental health, you can also practice intermittent fasting. Studies have found that with short-term fasting, people can significantly improve their everyday mood, tranquility, alertness, and even the feeling of euphoria. Not only that but also the symptoms of severe depression can be improved with fasting.

Treat or Prevent Disease

While we cannot guarantee that intermittent fasting will prevent you from developing a disease or treat an infection you already have, many studies have proven that fasting can help. These studies have shown that fasting a person can manage their symptoms, possibly reverse the condition, and significantly reduce your likelihood of ever developing a disease. Now that we have looked at the general ways in which intermittent fasting can improve your health, let's have a look at some of the specific diseases and conditions you can expect short-term fasting to improve.

Polycystic Ovary Syndrome (PCOS)

One common condition that affects women around the world, and the most prevalent of the endocrine disorders, is polycystic ovary syndrome. Though, you may know of this condition as the abbreviated PCOS. This condition causes a myriad of symptoms, such as fatigue, obesity, menstrual irregularity, infertility, insulin resistance, body hair, and more. These symptoms can only worsen as a woman age and go through menopause. Yet, despite how it affects the lives of so many women, doctors have to pinpoint the cause of this disorder. So far, it is only believed that genetics, insulin resistance, and excessive chronic inflammation can all contribute to the development and progression of this disorder.

While much still needs to be learned about both this disorder and its treatment, controlled scientific studies have revealed that intermittent fasting can greatly improve a person's life with PCOS. These studies have shown that when a woman practices regular short-term fasting paired with healthy nutrition, she can experience an improvement in many symptoms.

It is worth mentioning that the ketogenic diet has also been shown to be an especially helpful treatment option for women with PCOS, meaning that when you combine this diet with intermittent fasting, you can expect to improve your symptoms even further. In the studies on the ketogenic diet, it was found that not only did intermittent fasting improve overall symptoms, but previously infertile women were able to conceive.

Non-Alcoholic Fatty Liver Disease

A common condition in people who have developed excessive body fat, especially when located around the abdomen, is non-alcoholic fatty liver disease. The treatment of this disease is frequently weight loss, which, as you are now well aware of intermittent fasting is ideal for. However, the benefits of intermittent fasting for those with this form of liver disease go beyond just weight loss. After all, while it is most common for people with excessive abdomen fat to develop this disease, a person doesn't even have to be overweight to improve it. This disease is caused when fat builds up in the liver, but for some people, fat will build up in this organ even when they are at healthy body weight, making it even harder to treat. Yet, when fatty liver disease is left untreated, it leads to deteriorating health and may also develop into dangerous liver failure, which requires liver transplantation if the person is to survive.

Intermittent fasting can help because it not only helps you to reduce weight and, therefore, the importance of your liver but also because it changes how your body stores its fat. Through studying fatty liver disease, researchers found that individuals who are more prone to storing fat in their liver also have lower levels of a specific protein gene. The good news is that they also found intermittent fasting increases this protein gene, meaning that your liver is less likely to hold onto fat and more likely to shed excess weight. This can help both people who are currently seeking to rid themselves of non-alcoholic fatty liver disease and those who hope to prevent it in the future.

Diabetes

A person who is experiencing severe diabetes and having to undergo insulin treatment may be unable to practice intermittent fasting. Only your doctor will be able to determine whether or not you can safely practice short-term fasting. But, if your condition isn't as severe and your doctor believes it to be safe in your circumstance, then you will be happy to know studies have found intermittent fasting to be incredibly beneficial. Even if you cannot at this time practice intermittent fasting, you may still be able to improve your health enough through the ketogenic diet, at which time you could also take up intermittent fasting under your doctor's discretion.

As you know, intermittent fasting treats excessive weight gain, insulin resistance, and high blood sugar, so it is clear to see why it would help treat diabetes, which is characterized by these three occurrences. Intermittent fasting is so successful that one recent study even found that it was highly effective for type diabetes II patients who were reliant on insulin injections. The participants in this study practiced their fasting closely under their doctor's care multiple times a week. After a short time following their fasting schedule, they were able to completely reverse their insulin resistance, manage blood sugar levels, reduce excess body weight, and even stop their medication.

Alzheimer's Disease

Something that many of us begin to worry about as we age, especially if we have seen relatives go through it in the past, is Alzheimer's disease. This devastating disease not only separates family members in death but also in life. It separates a person from their very understanding and memory of themselves. Sadly, the rate of people with Alzheimer's disease has only continued to skyrocket over the past few decades, with it now being the sixth leading cause of death. The numbers have risen so much that, between the years 2000 and 2015, the rate of people increased by a shocking one-hundred and twenty-three percent, and it is only continuing to rise.

Sadly, science still does not have an answer on how to stop or reverse the disease. However, it has been shown that intermittent fasting can reduce a person's risk of developing it and lessen the severity. A large part of the reason that intermittent fasting is successful is that Alzheimer's disease consists of a mitochondrial cell dysfunction, although it has many other facets as well, such as dysfunctions in the immune system, protein genes, brain cells, and more. When these dysfunctions occur, it causes plaque to buildup in the neurofibrillary of the brain, causing oxidative stress, excessive chronic inflammation, and further mitochondrial dysfunction. It is a vicious cycle where the symptoms continuously cause the disease to worsen, which in turn makes the symptoms also worsen.

The many components of Alzheimer's disease lead to the brain's neurons becoming insulin resistant, and when they are no longer able to absorb the glucose needed, they can also no longer fuel the cells, leading to cellular starvation and death. But as intermittent fasting repairs mitochondrial cells and increases them in number, it can increase the number of cells able to fuel off of non-glucose fuels. It can also treat the insulin resistance itself and cause the production of ketones to fuel the non-mitochondrial neural cells.

Cancer

Lastly, studies have found that intermittent can reduce your likelihood of developing cancer and help make treatment more successful. As you are aware, intermittent fasting can help treat oxidative stress and cellular damage, both of which cause cancer. By reducing this damage, you can thereby reduce your risk of developing cancer in the future.

But that is not all. While human studies still need to be conducted, a study on mice found that when practicing short-term fasting chemotherapy treatment becomes more successful in targeting and treating both breast cancer and skin cancer. Not only did the chemotherapy itself become more effective, but the mice' immune systems also were better able to fight off the cancerous cells and growths, which is essential as chemotherapy is well-known for reducing a person's immune system drastically.

Chapter 11: Life-Changing Tips for Weight Loss Success

Losing weight does not mean following a diet for a few weeks and then giving yourself back to crazy joy. To really lose weight you need to identify what are your wrong habits, change them and maintain them over time, even after reaching the goal. If you do not change your lifestyle, the lost pounds will recover easily and in a short time you will return to the point you were before, with a 'yo-yo' effect that never ends.

1 - Do sports, the one that suits you best

Everyone tells us to exercise to lose weight. It is very true, but which and how? Maybe you could try Zumba: it is an aerobic sport, which allows you to consume several calories while having fun, but you have to see if it is suitable for your constitution. Physical activity must be customized according to your conditions: if for some prolonged aerobic work, such as step, running or Zumba, will be suitable, for others short and more intense work will be indicated, for others it will be important to work first on muscle mass, with weights and tools, and then on weight loss. Always evaluating the level of training and any problems, for example in the back or knees. In short, sport is an integral part of the lifestyle of those who want to lose weight and maintain a healthy weight, but at least in the beginning it is good to rely on an expert.

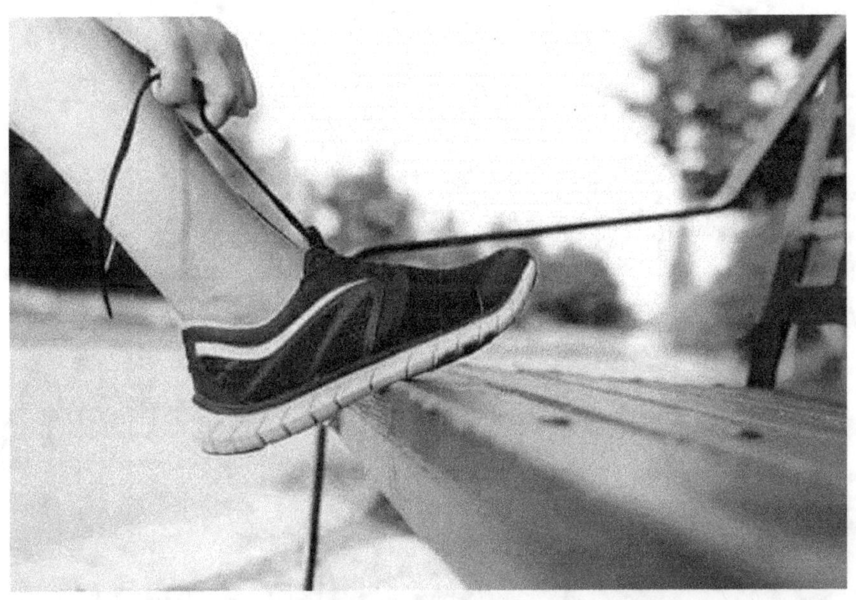

2 - Attention to the scale. Losing weight means losing fat

Losing weight doesn't just mean losing weight, but losing fat. If the needle of the scale goes down, it may be that we have only lost water or even muscle mass, which happens easily when doing a highly low-calorie diet. True, in the mirror you can see yourself a little slimmer and more deflated, but it is an apparent and not very long-lasting weight loss. For this reason, especially if the pounds to lose are several, it would be useful to rely on a serious professional, who in addition to getting us on scale measures the circumferences of certain critical points, determines body composition (fat mass, lean mass, percentage of water) through tests such as bio impedancemetry and evaluate the results of a diet over time.

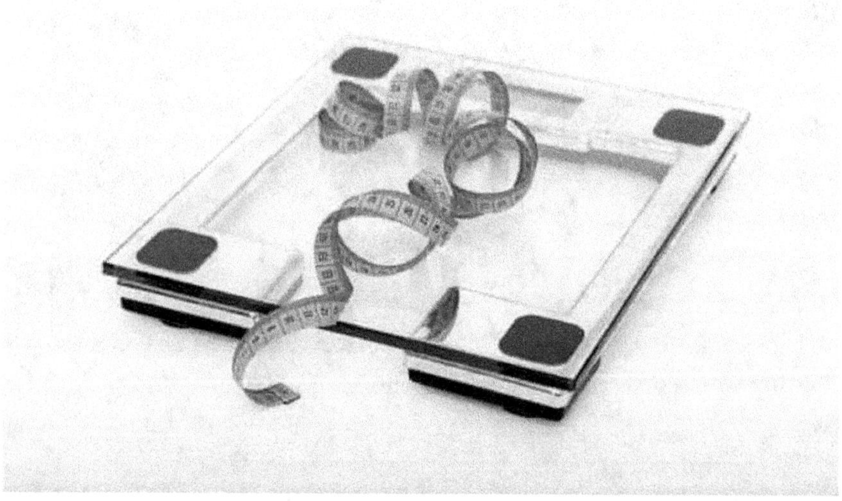

3 - Learn to read labels when shopping

Those who want to lose weight must acquire a food culture, and this means first of all reading the labels of what you buy and not just trust advertising. For example, if a product is defined as whole, the whole grain must be at the top of the list of ingredients; in a food that prides itself on being 'lean', fats cannot be second.

4 - One calorie is not the same as another

A tomato ripened in summer sun contains the same calories as a greenhouse tomato, but the former is much richer in micronutrients that not only are good for the body, but have a greater satiating and slimming reflex power; ditto for white and whole wheat flour, good quality oils and hydrogenated vegetable fats. The body cannot say 'I lack zinc or selenium', but it says 'I am hungry': if food supplies nutrients it needs, it receives satisfaction, otherwise it will be brought to look for more food. Too much caloric food with poor quality ingredients is poorly nutritious, not very filling and therefore provides empty calories. Therefore, for the same number of calories, effect on brain of food can be different. Following the seasonality and changing the food is also essential to avoid monotony, which is one of the reasons that push us to abandon diets.

5 - No to high-protein diets, but proteins are important

If it is true that high-protein diets are unbalanced, it is important, on the other hand, to ensure adequate protein intake. The protein is essential for maintaining muscle mass, stimulating the metabolism to 'burn', having a good tone, both physical and mental, feeling more efficient. A healthy person needs on average 1 gram of protein per pounds of body: for a woman of 143 lb. this means for example a handful of dried fruit (it is also allowed in diets, just do not overdo it!) Or an egg in the morning, a steak or a plate of pasta and legumes for lunch and a little fish in the evening.

6 - Choose the right fats

They are always demonized, instead according to the latest guidelines they must represent 25-30% of the daily income. Fats are precursors of hormones, that is, they serve to balance our endocrine system so they should not be abolished even when following a diet. And they serve all types of fats, as long as they are of quality: more than half of the daily requirement should come from monounsaturated fats, mainly from extra virgin olive oil, while the remaining part should be made up of equal parts of saturated fats, such as butter and the other fats of animal origin, and polyunsaturated, that is omega 6 contained in seed oils and omega 3, contained in blue fish and walnuts. Our body is perfectly able to metabolize fats, just avoid fried and fried foods, increase physical activity and drastically reduce simple sugars, which are the effective culprits of fattening. Finally, fats give flavor to the foods, make the diet more pleasant and compatible with family cuisine. Remember that no food makes you lose weight or gain absolute weight, it depends on how much you eat it and how it combines with other foods during the day.

7 - Avoid artificial sweeteners

It has been shown by several scientific works that artificial sweeteners, far from making you lose weight, contribute to fattening. The problem is not given by the amount of calories (which is zero in sweeteners) but by the signal that reaches the body. The sweet taste of sugar as well as sweeteners activates signals in the brain that push for more sugar and other food, with the result that we tend to eat more at the next meal. Studies from 2013 also showed that artificial sweeteners cause an alteration of glucose metabolism similar to that of diabetics, since they favor the transformation into fat of what he ate. As if that wasn't enough, another study from the same year found that saccharin and acesulfame, 2 of the most common sweeteners, block lipolysis, that is the mechanism that allows us to dissolve fats. In short, one could say that they make you more fat than lose weight.

8 - Avoid fructose

We are not talking about fructose naturally contained in fruit and vegetables, but fructose as an industrial sweetener, for example the corn syrup. Until recently it was thought that, having a lower glycemic index than sugar, it made you gain less weight. Controversy, fructose has a so-called preferential pathway of metabolism, which increases triglycerides and inflammatory levels of the liver which significantly interfere with weight loss. Already since 2004, scientific work had shown that fructose, taken continuously, increases insulin resistance like sugar and facilitates the onset of diabetes and metabolic diseases, such as obesity, while a 2013 study has shown that corn syrup induces obesity and cognitive decline, even favoring the development of diseases such as Alzheimer's. A damage that would already begin in the baby bump, because it seems that, if the expectant mother consumes fructose in large quantities, there is an activation of obesogenic mechanisms in the baby.

9 - Eat fruit, but don't drink industrial juices

It is one thing to eat a complete fruit, with its content of micronutrients and fibers that have satiating power, it is one thing to drink liters of juice which, even when they are 100% fruit, are deprived of the precious substances contained in the whole fruit. The fruit in a diet is welcome, but do not forget that it is still sugary, especially if we are talking about grapes, bananas or figs. But even fruits made up largely of water such as watermelon cannot be defined as 'slimming': a nice snack is refreshing, remineralizing and detoxifying, but you cannot eat half a watermelon instead of lunch in the illusion of losing weight!

10 - Dark chocolate is good, but not a whole bar

What about common belief that chocolate makes you lose weight? First of all we distinguish pure cocoa from chocolate. Cocoa has undisputed beneficial properties, is protective for the liver, contains precious and healthy polyphenols, and substances that can activate determine lipolytic mechanisms, but we are talking about pure bitter cocoa. Chocolate, on the other hand, is a delicious dessert that contains sugar and cocoa butter, which bring a lot of calories. Goodbye chocolate then? No: a square of good quality dark chocolate with at least 75-80% of cocoa fits perfectly, even in a weight loss diet, but not a bar of milk chocolate!

11 - Eat calmly and chew well

Hands up who has never eaten standing or in front of TV, PC and smartphone. On the other hand, if you want to lose weight, you have to look at it, smell it, savor it, chew it slowly. Keep in mind that already during chewing a series of signals are activated that arrive at the satiety centers of the brain, while the first blood signals arrive after 20 minutes, when they begin to absorb certain nutrients. If you eat quickly, you run the risk of finishing a whole meal before you realize you are full! Not only that: eating slowly allows you to gradually dilate the stomach, better assimilate what you eat, digest it more easily and better empty the intestines. If you chew badly, whole pieces of food arrive in the stomach, which require more intestinal work, with fermentations and swelling.

12 - Studying: makes you lose weight if you combine sport

That studying makes brain work and that activating the brain increases glucose consumption is true, but from here to say that studying makes you lose weight ... you should study walking! Instead, not only do you sit down, but you often fall into temptation to munch on something. In short, studying can make you lose weight if during the afternoon you have the opportunity to disconnect with an hour of sports, otherwise it is useless to delude yourself! I continually see people who join the gym to lose weight and then don't go there. Why? Because they didn't want to go at the start. Choose an activity suitable for you, whether it is swimming, dancing, fitness and martial arts and concentrate on that. Moving must give you the energy, the right energy to face the hour to dedicate to it, if already at the start what you have to do is not fun you will be able to spend 1 hour of physical activity without effort. Think carefully about which exercise you like best, many women prefer wear headphones with their favorite music and even walk for 2 hours without realizing it, others prefer to run, others prefer to dance. If you also like to move dancing know that on the web there are many Zumba videos that might be right for you, choose 3 or 4 and dance! Ditto regarding the jump with the rope or the ups and downs of the stairs of your apartment building ... any movement is good, if you find what you like *DO IT!*

13 - Don't shop when you're hungry

In fact, if you go shopping on an empty stomach, you risk buying a lot of junk food! When you go shopping instead, you need to go with a list of healthy foods that are part of the diet, staying away from the shelves of ready meals, chips and various sweets! Better to eat something before going to the supermarket or, in any case, not to feel the pangs of hunger. You will go home with bags full of everything except healthy food for your diet.

14 - Learn to read labels

You must always read the labels and therefore the ingredients to be sure of what you are buying. Reading ingredients very often it turns out that the food you intend to consume is not really healthy. The label of each product represents its *DNA*. Food often hides health pitfalls and the only way to defend yourself is to learn to read the label, which is an identity card of what comes to the table!

15 - Sleep about 7 hours a night

A good rest helps burn calories did you know? So take some time to relax before bed and then promote sleep: walk, read, take a nice relaxing bath and drink a purifying herbal tea. Sleeping well affects the effects of the weight loss diet and it is therefore clear that sleeping too little makes you fat, sleeping badly or not enough causes - after only a few days - increase in appetite hormones, leptin and ghrelin, and consequently the desire to eat.

16 - Drink minimum 8 glasses of water a day

Not only does it help you to purify yourself and therefore deflate you, but if you drink it before meals it helps you to reach a sense of satiety first. Avoid coke, wine, beer, sugary and sparkling drinks because they inflate and bring unnecessary calories. Drink lots and lots of water and often. Not only does it make a lot of urine and thus dispose (hopefully) that unsightly orange peel that reigns on your thighs, but it also speeds up your metabolism and makes you lose weight. Drinking water activates those metabolic mechanisms of heat production with energy expenditure. This would really help you lose weight. So drink a lot and drink often, and if it is difficult for you, I know many people who find it difficult to "drink" away from the table, at least in the morning treat yourself to a nice glass of water and lemon, already a good start to hydrate, detoxify and re-mineralize in a natural way!

17 - Use smaller dishes

It has been shown that we can "deceive" hunger simply by using smaller plates and glasses so why not do it? Focus on colors, take very colorful dishes, colors bring joy, turn the home shops or the markets, look for dishes smaller than those you used to use at home, there are also some reliable online stores such as Amazon where you can buy them without spending too much, get a flat plate, a deep plate and a dessert plate, you won't need to buy the full service

18 - Wake up your metabolism and always keep it active

How do you wake up your metabolism and keep it active all the time? Simple, first of all *THE MOVEMENT*, never do the diet without moving, the diet alone will work a little bit then we will stall. Second thing *EAT!* Snacks are important to make the thyroid work constantly. Even if you are not hungry but 3 hours have passed since the previous meal, eat something, be it yogurt, 2 rusks with fruit juice etc. Do not fast, *NEVER SKIP MEALS*, if the metabolism stops, it will also stop slimming.

19 - Don't be in a hurry

Hurry is known, it is the worst enemy of diet! Know that just as the pounds did not accumulate in one day, they will not magically go away in one night. Females and males body tends to retain the accumulated fat as a survival strategy and it takes time to reverse this course. Being impatient will also mean abandoning the diet immediately when the needle is not dropped. A good weight loss regimen must become a daily habit that we get used to over time and that will allow us to lose weight slowly and healthily. Many of these tips I am sure you already knew, but it is one thing to know them, another is to put them into practice, doing it will be simple, set a goal and do everything you can to achieve it, do you know what another excellent advice could help you? To *FILL A FOOD DIARY DAILY!*

20 - Fill in the food diary

In fact, writing down everything you eat during the day, starting from breakfast until dinner, is a valid way to correct mistakes and to understand what, how much and why you eat. The food diary should be a possibly not too large notebook, so that you can put it in your bag. The diary must be completed for at least 1 week, noting everything you eat and drink during the day, without neglecting any "rudeness". Close to the food we consume, we must enter the time, the quantity, the place where it was consumed, whether at home, at the bar, etc., the type of cooking and emotion that accompanied the snack, joy, nervousness, etc. Notes must be made when the food is consumed, in order not to forget anything. In this way, you can realize how many calories you consume. For example, breakfast apparently seems rather simple, on the contrary, it is rich in saturated fat. The same also applies to other meals eaten during the day.

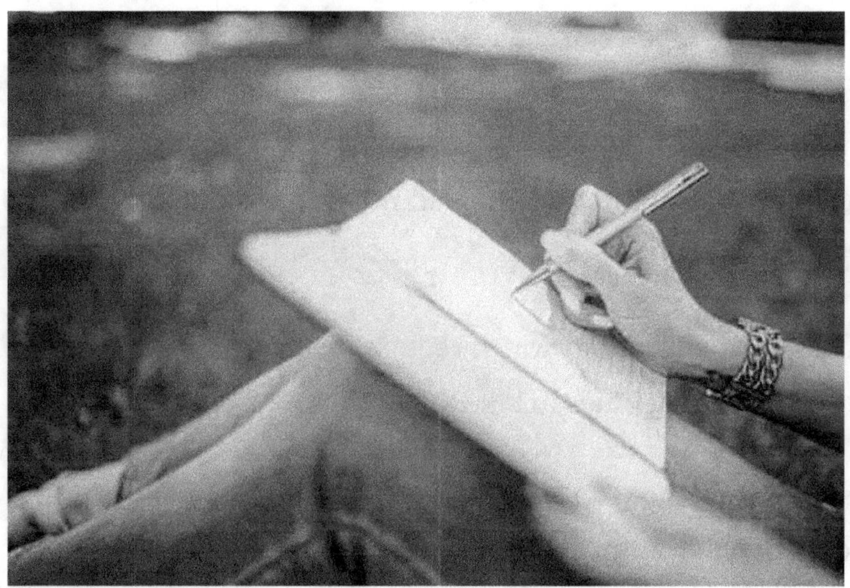

Chapter 12: Mostly Asked Questions and Answers on Intermittent Fasting

How long will I continue to fast?

Did you know that there are many commonalities between this feeding system and how naturally slender people eat? Some days they eat other times they just miss meals, that's how the nutrition is. If you become familiar with your selected IF schedule, your calorie intake will decrease until it becomes normal for you. You can change your frequency once you get the weight you need. It's best to keep fasting and not stop at all. It aims to permanently change your lifestyle, not just for a short time. It is a daily practice that guarantees consistent weight reduction.

I take some medications which require me to eat, what do I do during the fasting times to take the medicine?

You can experience some side effects when you take any medicines on an empty belly. Iron supplements can cause sickness and nausea; aspirin can cause stomach ulcers and upsets. It's better to ask the doctor if you should take this drug as you continue a fast. You can take the medicine with small, low-calorie leafy vegetables that do not interfere with your pace. Your blood pressure can drop over the fasting period so that if you take blood pressure-lowering medicine, the blood pressure may become too low and lead to headaches.

What food is better to eat raw or cooked vegetables?

There have been several discussions on this subject. Some argue that food preparation leads to vitamins, enzymes, and minerals destruction. But it also makes cellulose fiber more available for your system, among other nutrients. When prepared, carrots, fungi, spinach, chips, and other peppers, other vegetables provide more antioxidants, but the disadvantage is that Vitamin C may be lost when cooking. There is no official response; all you have to do is eat plenty of vegetables in whatever way you want.

I am old, is it too late for me to start fasting?

Starting fasting can never be too late. It can help you manage your appetite, help you lose weight, and even make your life longer. You'll quickly notice the impacts; you'll feel healthier, slimmer, and stronger. Start immediately.

When I take a treat like a packet of chips during my fasting period, what's going to happen?

Fasting is an intermittent activity involving voluntary meal abstinence. Not only does it help you, because you consume fewer calories, it's also because that's what your flesh was built to do. Do not equate fasting with starvation because starvation is bad, but fasting is good. IF's aim is to provide your body with free time to relax from food. Your improvement will end with just one snack and your blood sugar levels will allow you to get out of a fasted state.

What should I do if I don't lose weight?

Weight loss is a gradual process that takes quite some time to accomplish thus patients and consistency are needed. If you don't lose some weight in the first few weeks you should just keep going, you shouldn't be concerned. If you're going for an even longer period of time and still don't lose weight, it's wise to review what you eat as this is the most likely cause of the problems you might have. It's important to keep track of the food you eat so you can track the problem easily.

During my period, is it really safe to fast?

Fasting is not at all right when you are pregnant or breastfeeding, but your monthly cycles will not affect your fast in any way unless they are very painful or intolerable. If so, you can test your iron levels and take supplements as well.

 I have diabetes, can I still practice IF?

If you have type 1 or type 2 diabetes or on diabetes medication you need to take additional care while practicing IF. If the need arises, your doctor will check your blood sugar levels carefully to change your medicine prescription to allow them to co-exist with intermittent fasting peacefully. When you can't be closely monitored, don't attempt fasting. It decreases the blood sugar levels and continuing to take drugs as insulin can lead to exceptionally low concentrations of blood glucose that lead to hypoglycemia. You can drink a sugar-filled drink like soda and even stay off your fasting routine one day to raise the level of blood sugar. If you have blood sugar levels that are excessively low, this is due to over-medication and not intermittent fasting. Reduce your use of medications in advance because you expect lower levels of blood sugar when you begin IF.

Is it true that I can eat all I want on non-fast days?

This is true as all foods are allowed. It is permissible to use anything from the most oil-drenched fried chicken to a vegetable salad for any other meat. It is best not to consume too much as if during the time you were fasting you are struggling to eat what you would have. You may even overcome the impacts of fasting when you overfeed. It should not be made into a ritual of overeating after fasting, eating should be done responsibly. But it all boils down to what you want to do as you are the one that decides to fast and by now you already know a lot of the do and don't. You'll automatically find yourself choosing healthier meals after doing the fasting for some time.

Can I get tired from fasting, if so, how could I stop it?

No, the opposite would actually happen. Individuals have more strength in fasting as a result of higher levels of adrenaline in the body. With more than enough energy, you will certainly be able to conduct your ordinary operations. Fatigue is not a normal part of fasting, so if you feel extremely exhausted, stop fasting right away and see a doctor right away.

Can I receive the same benefits of fasting as an adult of the opposite sex?

Hormonally and metabolically, there are several differences between men and women. For example, women store more fat and are more susceptible to exercise-dependent fat burning. Research has shown that fasting females respond more quickly to endurance exercise while fasting males react more quickly with a weighted workout. IF's benefits on both genders are almost equal. It's not supposed to be a race, but more of individual experience, so concentrating on your body is better than thinking about others.

During the first days of fasting, I want to use meal replacement shakes, is it all right or should I just stick to food?

During the first days of IF training, these meal replacement shakes have helped most individuals. These are definitely better than calorie counting, as you can just sip free from your thirst. Even if the real nutrition is considered to be more effective when you like these drinks, you can go ahead and use them. Make sure that you only have those that have small or even no glucose.

Can I get the intermittent fasting result in me getting headaches?

Sure, but it only happens due to fatigue and not due to inadequate calories. You may have withdrawal symptoms, but they are gentle. Make sure you take medication on an ongoing basis to treat the migraine as you would a normal one. If during the fasting period you feel ill you must stop immediately.

If I observe intermittent fasting, what amount of weight can I lose?

That's based on a number of factors and variations between individuals. Such factors are like your heart rate, your exercise level, and how closely you observe the pace. During the first week, you will lose water and you will eventually lose weight as a result of your daily calorie intake. It's not advised to lose really fast weight and shouldn't be an aim, it's better to lose a little weight continuously.

Could I easily get cranky as I practice IF?

It has been used in all hundreds of years; this has never been an issue; it is not even in societies that have fasting as an essential part of their beliefs. Moreover, Buddhist monks are considered to be very peaceful people while they practically fast daily, fasting has no such effect.

I happen to be naturally slender thus I don't require any weight loss, can still practice IF for its physiological benefits?

If you're comfortable with your weight that's fine, fasting is very much still an option you have to improve your health. You have to make sure that during your feeding time you focus more on calorie-dense meals. Most slender people who fast get all the advantages without any problem. Testing through trial and error is the only way you can find the right balance between eating and fasting to keep you at a safe weight. Reduce the days of fasting by constantly checking your weight and take care not to get underweight as that would be hazardous to you.

Can I get too much food as a result of fasting?

The answer is yes and no to this question. First, it's really because you're going to consume more than you usually do after fasting. It is not, however, since feeding above the regular amounts in no days of fasting is not a consequence of fasting.

I'm going to sleep hungry when my fasting time is at night?

It's not probable, but it's mainly dependent on your metabolism, just try to keep your mind away from food and feel hungry. When you get out of your bed you may not feel hungry at all. Essentially, your appetite and hunger will suit your fasting routine.

Can IF make my body go into starvation mode to prevent more loss of fat?

This is not a realistic side effect because there is no calorie restriction on IF. There's no IF routine that's intense to the point you're going into starvation mode. The fasting time is short, so from the fat stores, the body absorbs fat and retains muscle mass. Research has shown that IF does not lower any individual's metabolic rate. Despite long fasts like those for three days, there will be no decrease in the basal metabolic rate. There is also no increase in the hunger hormone called ghrelin during IF.

I'm an overweight fellow, is IF really the key to solving my problem?

Intermittent fasting has proved to be one of the most effective and enduring strategies for obese individuals to lose and retain new weight. The bigger you are, the greater the initial loss of weight. You've most likely given up conventional restrictive diets. Intermittent fasting has an advantage over all of them because it is more versatile and when you consume anything it is not a crime because nothing is restricted. Research has shown that obese individuals are very easily used to fasting.

Can I eat during my fasting time if I really have to like during celebrations and major ceremonies?

Be active, but concentrate on what you're ingesting. While it's vital to get help from your family and friends, if you keep telling them you can't eat as you are in a fast, they'll start to get tired of hearing that and eventually you'll feel self-conscious. This will render it an obstacle to your normal activity, which is not its original intent, rather than something that fits perfectly in your life. When you know that there is a social event connected to food, then fast the day before or the day before. It is a very flexible device and without any difficulties you will continue to be active and enjoy these times.

Is low blood sugar an IF problem?

If your heart, which is a very powerful device, is stable, you can easily control blood sugar levels. When you obey the intermittent fasting guidelines in this book, your blood glucose levels must stay at a good level. If you are fasting for more than 2 days a week, the 24-hour fast technique is recommended.

Remember; always see a doctor before any major dietary changes

I decided to get pregnant, should I keep on fasting?

This issue has not been widely studied but it is not understood whether IF has an effect on fertility in so far. Fertility may be affected by other extremely intense types of fasting. If you're trying to get pregnant, stop fasting to be on the good side of things, but note that once you do fast, it's absolute restrictions as you may risk the unborn child.

Conclusion

A healthy diet can be overwhelming, especially when it comes to shifting from a typical western diet of fast foods and sugar-loaded treatments. Being over 50 doesn't make it any easier. Nonetheless, after a few weeks on the fasting regiment, you will see an improvement in your mind, what you feel about yourself, your body and your life in general. Most individuals claim they have a lot of energy after practicing fasting for just a week or two. If you are overweight and have a high percentage of body fat, you'll love the first week since you'll lose the most weight in that period. More importantly, with regular exercise, you will feel better and sleep better. It is going to do so much more than make you look slimmer and feel more comfortable. These will add to your general health and can help avoid the many nutrition-related diseases and conditions that you are seeing today. So, when you're distracted by old eating habits or sometimes hunger, catch a healthy snack or re-read the encouragement tips in this book, take a long walk and ask a buddy to meet you for one of your planned treats. Consider why you do this and celebrate the way you look and sound that can give you the lifts you need to conquer those obstacles on the path to better well-being.

The journey to an effective fasting system can be very challenging. Here are some domain navigation laws. Taking things one step at a time to understand the implications of the plan. Gradually pursue the method of fasting. You don't just want to move for something that may not be for you without thinking. You will continue fasting once every three weeks until you slowly change the time limit as you wish. For everyone, no one system works the same way. Choose a scheme and configure it to suit your needs.

Decide whether it's good for you. Even after considering its many positive benefits, note that IF is not for everyone. The knowledge of nutrition and exercise will decide whether you can pursue it. If you are new to fitness and food, I strongly recommend that you first recognize the basics. Start slowly, smoothly, and gradually. If you decide you'd like to try IF, there's no rush. Pick one specific thing to try, even if it's a regular meal change of just one hour. Try this out and see how it works for you. Reflect on what IF strategies have in common, instead of going into too much detail. Sometimes you're feeding and sometimes you're not doing it that almost sums it up.

Remember what's happening in your life Consider about how much preparation you're doing and how intensively you're practicing, how well you're going to rest and heal, how well IF blends into your daily practice or normal private activities, and what other stresses or life needs include. Note IF this feature is one of the many forms of diet. But it is best only when it is regular, elastic, and part of your normal practice, not a task, and not a persistent physical and psychological pain source.